Image of the cattle sector and its products

Image of the cattle sector and its products

Role of Breeders Association

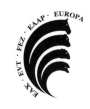

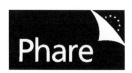

Editor:

Jean Boyazoglu

EAAP Technical Series No. 4

CIP-data Koninklijke Bibliotheek, Den Haag

ISBN 9076998337
ISSN 1570-7318
paperback

Subject headings:
Animal registration
Animal identification
Breedeers' Association

First published, 2003

Wageningen Academic Publishers
The Netherlands, 2003

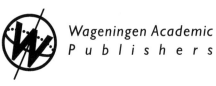

Wageningen Academic
P u b l i s h e r s

Table of content

Preface

Preface

Three basic factors: safety, quality and the way in which the product is produced determine behaviour of consumers and their choice of food products. This is particularly true for the cattle sector and its products, whose image was seriously affected by outbreaks of two major cattle diseases in the recent past.

How to improve the image of the sector and its products was the main theme that gathered over 110 participants from eleven European countries, eight of which were, at that time, candidates for the membership in the European Union at the workshop organised within the BABROC project[1]. The workshop also discussed possible trends in the cattle sector in the new EU member countries. In addition to the number of participants, the workshop represented a specific event in the history of cattle breeders associations in Europe. It was a forum at which the highest EU authorities declared their full support to the European cattle industry and to the efforts of cattle producers to improve the image of the sector and to regain the consumer's confidence.

Breeder's associations from then EU candidate countries being aware of the fact that the admission of their respective countries in the EU would bring new challenges and tasks to all segments of society, undertook a range of activities aimed at facilitating the integration of the cattle sector in the EU system. The BABROC project provided an excellent opportunity for officials and professionals from these associations to get acquainted with the *acquis communautaire* relevant to the cattle sector and with experiences and practices of associations from Austria, Germany and Italy, which also participated in the project. In addition, the project assisted associations from Central and Eastern European candidate countries to introduce new services to their members and to improve quality of the existing services.

Marketing of cattle products represents a major activity of associations of cattle breeders and cattle producers. In the recent past, consumption of cattle products, particularly consumption of beef, seriously declined both in the existing EU member countries and in the EU candidate countries, manly due to the effect of BSE and, later FMD outbreaks. Competent bodies of the European Union, national associations and national authorities undertook series of measures first, to eradicate diseases affecting the sector and, second, to assist producers in regaining consumers' confidence.

The first step was the introduction of a comprehensive system for identification and registration of cattle and of labelling of beef and beef products in 1997. This was followed by the application of the EU systems of Denomination of Protected Origin (DPO), Protected

---

[1] The project «Strengthening of **B**reeders' **A**ssociations as **B**usiness **R**epresentative **O**rganisations in **C**entral and Eastern Europe» - BABROC- was approved by the EU Phare Business Support Programme.

Image of cattle sector and its products

Geographic Indication (PGI) and Guaranteed Traditional Speciality (GTS) to cattle products, including the labelling of beef. All these measures are expected to provide for full information to consumers and to guarantee «traceability» of products from the farm to the table.

However, it is to be noted that the cattle producers are also confronted with the ambiguous position of consumers: while declaring concern for the way in which the product is produced, they often opt for cheaper products regardless of the way in which it is produced. This should not, in no way, impede or slow down efforts aimed at attaining the maximum of food safety and the highest possible quality of products.

For this reason, the workshop recommended the establishment of a European structure for the exchange of technical and commercial information among cattle breeders associations and for their joint work in improving safety, quality and the image of cattle industry and cattle products. The proposed future activities should also ensure the continuous flow of information from producers to consumers, as well as the feed back signals to producers. Improvements in the image of the cattle sector and its products in Europe require full participation and contribution of mass media as well as of specialised publications and programmes in electronic media.

Welcome address by Dr. Franz Fischler

Commissioner for Agriculture, European Commission, Brussels

Ladies and Gentlemen,

First I wish you good evening and thank you for the invitation to your conference. To this, I add a few brief reflections, since this should remain a welcome address. On the slate behind me I can see, that among other things your discussions were about the image of the cattle industry. I think that here, we must be very straight forward. What constitutes our image?

The first point is that there is the question of food safety, which played an enormous role in the last months and years. Therefore we must be frank and remember that our meat and other products of animal origin, which is by far the largest production sector of the European Union, have never been as safe as they are now. Thus, we have nothing to hide. The problem is, however, how to convey this message to the consumer? Sometimes, the opinion differs. Heated discussions on BSE and Foot and Mouth disease are responsible for this. In other words, I think that we must and you must do something, so that the good quality of our products becomes sufficiently known to the consumer.

The second thing that I would like to say, is that in my opinion for agricultural production quality will become more and more important in the future; for that we must be careful. We should not yield to those forces that want to create a standardized quality and Europe-wide regulations on what is quality and what is not. Food safety must be regulated. But still, I would like to decide which meat I like best, and I do not want prescriptions from anybody else. I think that most consumers are of the same opinion, and thus the market should be the decisive factor and those producers, that are prepared to produce the respective qualities, should get a chance in the market.

Third aspect is that today consumers, in fact most citizens, observe closely how a product is produced. Therefore, the ability to trace the origin of products is becoming a more and more important factor. The question how to produce is a question that is increasingly considered a component of quality. We should keep this development in mind. I am of the opinion that we should first take care that there are incentives for those who are interested in quality. We should also develop our joint agricultural policy in this direction and in connection with this we should affirm ourselves in the international market. What I mean with affirm ourselves? I think that we have no reason not to be offensive in the new round of the WTO. We should use our influence so that quality becomes more recognised in the international market, so that there are fair conditions, and above all, so that our politics take the quality of animal husbandry and animal welfare into account, so that they are secured at an international level. European farmers should not be punished because they have higher standards than others in the world.

1

Image of cattle sector and its products

These I think are the considerations that will be important in the near future. Apart from that we have several major tasks ahead of us. We have to see to it, that we achieve a sensible market-equilibrium in beef production, so that the too low market prices for beef rise again. We also must tell the consumers that they should not be ambiguous. One thing is certainly insupportable; a consumer who is shocked when he sees pictures on television where animals are treated badly or of chicken that live in cages, but who looks only at the price when he is in the supermarket, regardless of whether the eggs that he buys come from chicken freely roaming or from chicken in cages. This ambiguity makes life hard for farmers. We should also do something to improve our image and see to it that this ambiguity does not linger on.

In this spirit I wish you, as the people responsible in the animal farming sector, great success and I would like to congratulate EAAP and our Italian friends on the organization of this conference.

Thank you.

Speech by the Italian Minister for Agriculture, Mr. Giovanni Alemanno

What in my opinion should be underscored on the occasion of this meeting, in the presence of Commissioner Fischler, whom I thank for being here, is that the Italian cattle breeding sector, after paying too-high a price for the inefficiency and the malfunctioning of the Italian public administration system, may today begin to see the light anew, because we have finally started mechanisms and new procedures aimed at launching the Cattle Register by 1st June 2002.

Thanks to the new Internet technologies, we shall be in a position to offer all cattle breeders, administrators, and consumers the full traceability of heads of cattle, both beef and dairy. This will enable all the players concerned to focus on quality, appropriate cattle raising techniques, ensuring the latter's effectiveness, thus allowing sector operators to document, in a clear and reliable way, the origin and quality of their products. Thanks to the Internet, people shall be able to link directly to the new Cattle Register in order to obtain all types of information.

It will be open to all those wanting to surf our sites, or to get in touch with our reference bodies; a long negotiation phase has been accomplished, we have had to cope with considerable red tape, and answer the autonomy claims by the Regional Authorities which wanted to be granted their own control and management tasks over the regional Cattle Register; however we shall now have real-time data entry and reading.

A further aspect to be highlighted is that data entry in the cattle register shall not only be performed by public veterinaries, but also by the agricultural assistance centres belonging to professional associations and by cattle breeders associations, i.e. the various territorial realities of AIA. This choice was made in order to give credit to the association activities of breeders, as well as to their ability to create service centres such as the CAA (agricultural assistance centres).

Two directions must be followed in order to reform the public administration system: on the one hand enhancing the greater efficiency afforded by the new technologies, which provide a direct contact between citizens and the public administration, and on the other empowering the associations spread over the national territory by increasing their concrete and active participation in the management of the Register.

No doubt this new responsibility implies the need to increase the sanctions against those who do not comply with the rules, ensuring a greater and more alert presence by the officials in charge of controls. However, if we work together, we shall be able to ensure that never again the Italian cattle breeding sector's credibility is put in question owing to a few bad examples, nor that it finds itself, in case of serious crises such as the BSE outbreak, unprepared and incapable of ensuring specific guarantees to consumers, with serious and unfair financial consequences for cattle breeders.

In the past few weeks the first case of human BSE was identified in Italy: this is the result of a time-bomb situation which we have inherited from a distant past, after the long period of time elapsed between the consumption of infected meat, and the emergence of symptoms. However, we were deeply distressed by this contagion, which has endangered the life of a young girl. This shock has urged us to take a further commitment, that is that the control and assessment system, revitalised by a growing co-operation between the public administration and cattle breeders, is always to provide total certainty, also and with special reference to imports.

The future we are building with the Cattle Register, and thanks to the strengthening of the prevention system against BSE-related risks, is a future of clarity and transparency, the two features that will enable us to ensure the protection of the Italian cattle breeding sector, a very important one indeed, with a long history, and, more importantly, an extraordinary human resource heritage, made up of people who strongly believe in what they do.

In this connection, AIA is called to play an essential role, just as producers associations are, and we shall always act as to ensure that they participate in all choices, proposals, and projects to come. Thank you for your attention.

Presentation by AIA's Chairman, Mr. Nino Andena

Mr Minister, and Mr Commissioner, since it is getting late, and I was asked to stick to time limits, I shall pass over formal procedures.

Consequently, I shall briefly summarise what Babroc is, and the topics that were dealt with in greater detail during this meeting, whose session started this morning at 9 am.

Babroc is a community project promoted by EAAP, by means of which three EU Countries, namely Italy, represented by AIA, Germany, and Austria interact with other Eastern Europe Countries in order to carry out technical training and information initiatives, thus promoting osmosis and integration, in the light of the possible entry of these Countries into the European Union.

I would like to thank EAAP in particular, and Professor Boyazoglu for making this meeting come true, and for their invaluable contribution.

Today's meeting convened here in Verona the representatives of cattle breeders associations coming from most of Europe, and all the problems affecting this sector at this particular time in history have been dealt with.

Two issues were particularly focused by debate:
- milk quota restrictions
- methodologies to cope with animal health and healthiness emergencies, i.e. the issue of BSE, which brought about a slump in production in the dairy sector, and caused a crisis in the meat sector.

The different aspects at stake have been identified, and a great number of indications have emerged with reference to the common actions to be implemented in order to prepare for the enlargement of the European Union. Interesting, perhaps difficult actions, that have elicited agreement on many points, and that have highlighted those on which considerable work remains to be done in order to achieve the goals set. However, what has emerged was the firm willingness to work together to meet our targets.

The cattle breeding selection system, today well represented here, represents, both in Italy and Europe, the core of all policies aimed at ensuring the future of European cattle breeding. Indeed, as stated in a book published with the Ministry's contribution, which I would like to present you, entitled «The Structure of Dairy Cattle Breeding in Europe and Italy»; 40% of the firms we managed to rejuvenate are aged between 35 and 40 years, and why, in the whole of Europe, while the number of cattle farms dwindles, this sector has gained increasing importance. So, cattle farms which are currently closing are those that do not participate in this system, whether they be in favourable areas, or in disadvantaged mountain locations.

Also breeders' satisfaction for the services provided by the association system is an indication of the future of European cattle breeding.

Image of cattle sector and its products

We have spoken of food safety, of the greater multifunctionality that the system must achieve, starting from its well-established operational prerequisites, represented by functional controls, and by its traditional book-keeping activity, by improving operations in terms of the provision of technical assistance, and of traceability systems.

During this meeting we have delved deeper into the labelling system established by AIA, a system approved by the Ministry, which is functioning perfectly, and that underscores the fact that the cattle breeding system has shifted its interests from a single task, that of functional controls, to a service multifunctionality not only tailored to benefit cattle breeders, but also the institutions, and, in particular, consumers.

From this meeting all the prerequisites for a re-launch of the sector may be extracted, a re-launch which we sorely need, both in the dairy and beef sectors.

The conditions are there to ensure that, by means of the adoption of certain guidelines, all sector operators, both those in the European Union, and in the Countries which are about to enter the Union, may face the future by reducing the current degree of uncertainty in the markets.

These certainties and guarantees are needed to an even greater extent by farming entrepreneurs. The expertise afforded by our services will no doubt take care of the rest.

Registration system in each EU country

J. Claus

*Association for Dairy Quality Control Lower Saxony
Grebenstr. 19, D27283 Verden, Germany*

Summary

Health is a fast growing concern of the human society. The stronger focus on health demands safe foods. Wheras formarly control was mainly concentrated on product control, today public control includes the individual animals from birth till slaughter.

The new control concept requires a unique identification system for all individual animals. Globalization of the industry and trade lead to the additional requirement of an international / world-wide compatible identification system.

Historically identification and registration of individual animals has been limited to the breeding part of a population. Different identification systems have been practiced, variing from colour description to double plastic eartags. Compatibility across countries and often within countries was not possible or in practice difficult to build up.

High requirements and the diversity of traditional identification systems led to the regulation Nr. 820 / 97 in which the EU introduced in 1997 a comprehensive system on „Identification and registration of cattle and labelling of beef and beef products».

Today all EU countries maintain a system for identification and registration according to the EU – regulation. It is possible to display centrally the complete life history of each individual.

In case of any disease or feedstuff problem it has been successfully proven to identify the animals related to the problem at short notice, wherever the animals are or have been kept or have been slaughtered.

Together with the beef labelling system today it is practiced to withdraw beef products from the stores "over night".

The EU – identification and registration systems has proven undoubtly as the key for a highly efficient veterinary control and consumer protection system.

Kurzfassung

Gesundheit ist ein schnell wachsendes Anliegen unserer heutigen Gesellschaft. Der stärkere Focus auf Gesundheit erfordert gesunde Nahrungsmittel. Während früher Kontrollen in erster Linie auf Produktkontrolle ausgerichtet war, schließen öffentliche Kontrollen heute das Einzeltier vom Geburtsstall bis zur Schlachtung ein.

Image of cattle sector and its products

Das neue Kontrollkonzept erfordert ein einheitliches Identifikationssystem für alle Tiere. Die Globalisierung der Industrie und des Handels führt zu der zusätzlichen Forderung nach einen international kompatiblen Identifikationssystem.

Historisch war die Identifikation und Registrierung der Rinder auf die Zuchtpopulation beschränkt. Unterschiedliche Identifikationssysteme wurden praktiziert, die von Farbebeschreibungen bis zu doppelten Plastikohrmarken reichten. Die Kompatibilitaet zwischen Ländern und oftmals auch innerhalb Länder war nicht gegeben oder in der Praxis schwer aufzubauen.

Hohe Anforderungen und die unterschiedlichen traditionellen Identifikationssysteme führten zur EU – Verordnung Nr. 820/97, in der die EU ein umfassendes System zur Identifizierung und Registrierung von Rindern und Etikettierung von Rindfleisch und Rindfleischprodukten einführte.

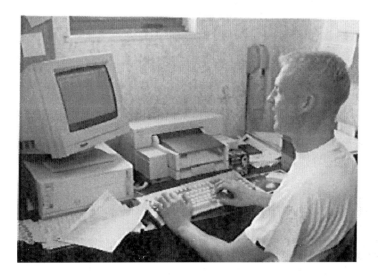

Electronic access to the national data bank for cattle registration

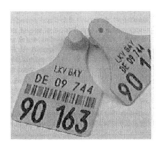

Eartags according to EU regulations

Reporting birthes by post cards.

Heute betreiben alle EU – Staten die Identifikation und Registrierung der Rinder nach den EU – Verordnungen. Die Registrierung schließt eine Speicherung aller Daten in einer nationalen Datenbank ein.

Im Falle von Seuchenausbrüchen oder anderen Veterinaerproblemen konnte erfolgreich gezeigt werden, daß Tiere sicher identifiziert und ihre Lebenswege zuverlässig aufgezeigt werden können.

Zusammen mit der Fleischetikettierung ist somit ein wirksamer Verbraucherschutz gegeben. Das EU – Identifikations- und Registrierungssystem hat sich zweifelsfrei als hochwirksames System für Veterinärkontrollen und Verbraucherschutz erwiesen.

1. Identification and registration as a part of a comprehensive control system

Questions like "which animal is it", "when and where was this animal born" "when and to which places has this animal moved" have been the concern since decades for veterinarians as well as for breeders and other agricultural bodies.

Until late 20th century in most countries individual cattle identification and registration has been restricted to animals under a control system for breeding and/or performance recording. The proportion of such animals relative to the total cattle population varied between countries between 20 to 80 %.

BSE with all it´s well known dramatic effects on control demands and loss of consumer confidence was a strong promotor for an EU – regulation on "Cattle Identification and Registration and Beef Labelling", first time released in 1997.

The scope of the system was and still is:

- Support of disease management and disease prevention
- Traceability of beef products from the store to the birthplace of the animals, and
- Control of farm subsidies based on cattle keeping

The main focus of these scopes are various control systems, based on a unique identification systems and a centralized registration system for the life history of the total cattle population.

2. History of cattle identification

Cattle identification has a history as long as breeding takes place. Initially, color description/painting was the tool for individual identification. Gradually in addition to color description or as substitute different numeric coding systems of animals have been introduced:

- Ear notching, brand marking, metal tags, plastic tags, and electronic tags.

Traditionally the design of tags has been different as well als the uniqueness of the coding/numbering systems was restricted to countries or even to organizations within countries.

The diversity of coding systems in addition to the limitation of identification to the active breeding part of the population made it impossible to unify or enlarge existing systems. An EU – wide complete new system for identification and registration was therefor the only solution to the specific veterinary challenge and consumer confidence situation caused by BSE.

3. EU – regulation on identification and registration

Intitially Cattle Identification and Registration has been defined in EU regulation 820 of 1997 and was updated in regulation 176 of 2000 under the title "System for the Identification and Registration of Bovine Animals and Labelling of Beef and Beef Products".

Concerning the identification and registration part, the regulations have 5 elements:

1. A coding system that ensures numeric uniqueness of animal and farm / holding identification across countries
2. Eartags in specified material and size
3. Central national electronic data bank with details on events and contents of reports/storage
4. Passports with data requirements for each animal leaving a farm / holding
5. Farmregister as a subset of the national data bank on farm / holding level.

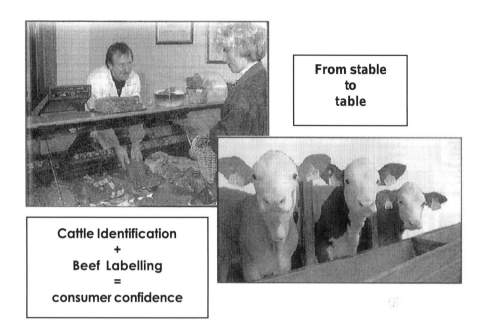

The overall concept of cattle identification an beef labelling.

The national data bank has to contain the complete actual cattle population with all it´s historic birthes, movements (within a country as well as imports and axports), and slaughters. Actuality of the national data bank is given through the request to report all events within 7 days.

4. Status in EU Countries

3 years after the release of the EU – regulation 370/1997, all countries have completed the requirements of this regulation or are near to completeness. Experience has shown, that the establishment of such a system is a huge logistic challenge with the demand for a clear organizational concept and a high financial budget.

5. Contribution of cattle identification and registration to recover consumer confidence

The succes of the establishment of an national systen for identification and registration system as required today by the EU may be seen from historic and present examples:

- At times *without national identification and registration:*
  It took weeks, to find the life history of the beef cow „Cindy» which was the first BSE – case in Germany.
  The search for the life history was escorted by week long discussions about deficits in public consumer protection.
- Nowadays *with national identification and registration:*
  Additional feedstuff was supposed (not proven) to be contaminated with antibiotics. Within hours after notice all possible affected animals have been be located and banned,
  beef products of possible affected animals was withdrawn from stores
- *Public notice*: There has been a problem with antibiotics in feedstuff, all necessary actions for consumer protection have been completed.

6. Conclusion

The EU – regulations for beef labelling based on a consistent animal identification and registration system is the key for a highly efficient veterinary control and consumer protection system. It supports the aim ti regain consumer confidence in agricultural products.

Specificity, DPO, PGI, traceability and labelling of beef

S. Cuore Catholic University, Piacenza, Italy

This paper is first of all focused on specificity of traditional food products, with particular attention to the products differentiated by EC Regulations 2081/92 and 2082/92, on their specific links with the territory and their impact on rural development. The second part is dedicated to the analysis of EC Regulation 1760/00 concerning beef labelling, especially to its utility for consumer information. Finally, reference is made to EC Regulation 178/02 concerning the interdependence between «labelling», «traceability» and food safety.

In questo lavoro si presenta in primo luogo le peculiarità dei prodotti tipici, ponendo particolare attenzione alle differenziazioni sottolineate dalle normative comunitarie EC 2081/92 e 2082/92, alla specificità del prodotto strettamente connesso con l'ambiente ed all'impatto sullo sviluppo rurale.

In secondo luogo viene analizzata la normativa comunitaria EC 1760/00, inerente l'etichettatura, con particolare attenzione sull'utilità dell'informazione al consumatore.
In fine andremo si presenta la normativa comunitaria 178/02 EC, ponendo l'accento sull'interdipendenza esistente tra l'etichettatura, la tracciabilità e la sicurezza alimentare.

1. Specificity, DPO, PGI and GTS

The European Commission initiated an investigation on rural development in 1988, with a communication to the Council and to the European Parliament entitled «The future of the rural world» (Com. (88) 501 def.), giving this subject a new importance for agricultural and structural politics in the European Union. Furthermore, amongst the tools used to face «the challenge of the rural world», is cited in the same document, as another novelty, the politics of quality for agro-food industry products.

However, it is only in 1992 that the McSharry reform on Agricultural Policy was approved, obtaining as a complementary measure the approval of two regulations, 2081 and 2082, with the consequent creation of a «Denomination of Protected Origin» (DPO), a «Protected Geographic Indication» (PGI) and a «Guaranteed Traditional Speciality» (GTS).

These two regulations introduced the tools to support the food and agriculture sector of the European Union that are not expressed into direct help payments for the farmers. Nevertheless, these are not less important; in fact their main objective is to protect those agro-food industry products that present peculiar features connected to the territory, the socio-economical and cultural environment that determine them. If in fact there is a strong and identifiable connection between a product's quality and the features of the territory where the product was obtained, protecting its production gives, as well, socio-economical support to those rural territories that knew how to preserve these products over time and are still able to offer them to the consumers. Therefore, the protection of these products represents a necessary condition for their further and progressive valorisation on bigger and more competitive markets, even if on its own it is certainly not a sufficient condition to obtain a secure commercial success and to promote the local development of the rural areas.

Besides, this agro-food industry production is very often collocated to difficult, sometimes marginal rural areas, or anyway in areas where because of territory conformation, space dislocation and climatic instability, or for any other structural justification, a mere competition based only on production costs cannot be considered. We thus understand better how the protection of these products can also contribute to sustain and promote the economical development.

Moreover, it is obvious that a quality product can have a «pulling» function for the entire economy of the area it is related to; it can be involved, besides the agricultural production activity, first of all with the transformation industry, but also the more commercial industries, *e.g.* tourism, entertainment, restaurants and spare time.

With the term «typical product» are generally intended agriculture and food products that are characteristic for their specificity when compared to similar products of different origin, because they were obtained in a certain environment, in well defined, and in some ways unique, pedological, climatic and exposure conditions, but also because of the existing production, cultural and environmental traditions.

Natural factors, *i.e.* the climate and the land's physical-chemical and morphological characteristics, contributed to determine some basic bonds for a local characterization of the production practices; some of these practices are, in fact, specific to a territory and not reproducible elsewhere. On the other hand the human factor, particularly its cultural component, has allowed for a specific territorial characterization of the production processes through the development of technologies that have improved through time following an evolution, always respectful of traditions. A typical food product can thus be considered as a result of creativity, with a typical historical aspect and a link to a specific region of origin. This specificity is strengthened by the strong interdependence existing between quality of the raw agricultural material and quality of the final product.

The local and ancient character of the series of operations that result in a typical food product is of special value from the point of view of the economy of quality. The latter character assigns to the product, besides its special degree of excellence and the value of its intrinsic properties to which it initially owes its renown, other qualities that are today of special value. In fact, the product's strong dependence to history and the territory collocates it in a system of society values that appreciate the product as well for other features, *i.e.* the strength of its link with nature, the tight dependence with production practices that do not leave space to «artificial treatments», the capacity to mobilize traditional resources and the incorporation in a region's rich gastronomic patrimony.

In other words, the strong quality-territory relation which links the differentiated product with a specific geographic origin is completely coherent with the main idea that assimilates quality with the capacity to satisfy specific needs. It is important to emphasize the rich meaning of the binomium history-territory, which confers to the typical product a series of features that are of special value and not reproducible by technology.

A recent survey carried out by *Eurobarometro* for the EU indicates that *«for 9 out of 10 Italians, the European Union should guarantee the quality of food products as a priority over the struggle against unemployment, poverty and crime»*. This survey emphasizes how the preferences expressed by the Italians «are contrary to what is indicated by the European media, which relegates food quality guarantee to the fifth position». These results confirm the obvious interest of Italians for good food, and attribute to our Country the responsibility to play a major first role in the European policy definition of food quality and safety.

Nevertheless, from a formal point of view, the two cited regulations only take into consideration typical products with a Denomination of Protected Origin (DPO), a Geographic Protected Indication (GPI) and a Traditional Guaranteed Speciality (TGS), therefore identifying only a part of the whole universe of typical products in general; the abovementioned «protections» are though becoming more and more important with the passing of time and with the growing list of products that have obtained a protection.

The EC regulation n. 2081/92 – relevant to the protection of denominations of origin and geographic indications of agriculture and food products[1] - requires the registration of products with a denomination of origin and a geographic indication. This registration

---

[1]Modified by the regulations (EC) n. 535/97 of the Council (GUCE n. L. 83 of March 25th 1997, p. 3), n. 1068/97 and n. 2796/2000 of the Commission (respectively in GUCE n. L. 156 of June 13th 1997, p. 10 and n. L. 324 of December 21st 2000, p. 26).

protects the products not only in their country of origin, but also on the whole territory of the European Union. In article 2, paragraph 2, of the regulation are defined the two categories of protected names:

1) *Denomination of origin:* the name of a region, of a specific place, or in exceptional cases of a country, designating an agriculture or food product:
    - Native to the region, the specific place, or country;
    - With a quality or characteristics due essentially or exclusively to the geographic environment, including natural and human factors, and whose production, transformation and elaboration takes place in the defined geographic area;

2) *Geographic indication:* the name of a region, of a specific place, or in exceptional cases of a country, designating an agriculture or food product:
    - Native to the region, the specific place, or country;
    - With a specific quality, status, or other characteristic, that can be attributed to the geographic origin, and whose production and/or transformation and/or elaboration takes place in the defined geographic area.

The EC regulation n. 2082/92 – relevant to the specificity of agriculture and food products - establishes a certification system for those agricultural products using traditional raw materials, or that have been obtained using a traditional production or transformation methods and are clearly differentiated from other similar products of the same category. Products with these qualifications can bear a European Community label and symbol underlining their specificity.

Article 2 of the regulation 2082/92 defines the notion of specificity as *«one or more elements that clearly distinguish an agriculture or food product from other products or foods that are part of the same category»*. It states that product presentation is not considered as an element according to the abovementioned definition, and furthermore that specificity cannot limit itself to the qualitative or quantitative composition, to the production method indicated in a European or national regulation, nor in the optional regulations established by normalisation organisms, unless this regulation has been elaborated to *define a product's specificity.*

Although they favour quality development, these regulations do not fix any objective rule of quality, instead they guarantee a product's origin and specificity and induce the consumers' quality expectations. Therefore these regulations only draw an outline, without giving mandatory indications on product quality. The definition of product quality is the task of the producer. Taken together, these two regulations fundamentally pursue three main objectives.

1. The development of regional productions and specialities to favour agricultural production diversification and contribute to the development of rural zones;
2. To offer a support to the commercial initiatives of the producers; such tools are made available not only to permit the producers to differentiate their products, but also to protect them from abuses or usurpations;
3. The consumers' protection; a reliable information about the product should be supplied as a priority to consumers that give importance to its origin or production method.

These objectives clearly underline two aspects: on the one hand, they contribute in the accomplishment of one of the largest goals of the PAC reform, *i.e.* to bring closer production and market requirements. On the other hand, these set objectives take into consideration the requirements of both consumers and producers. Only a system including both groups can match the interest of both parties and thus guarantee a lasting success.

The case here is to emphasise on the fact that the regulation relevant to the attestation of specificity represents a novelty compared to the national pre-existing arrangements, even compared with the dispositions of Member States regarding the so-called quality brands. Instead, the regulation on the protection of geographic indications and denominations of origin takes inspiration on the already existing autonomous initiatives of some Member States.

Nevertheless, the connection between typical product and territory varies a lot between the different types of protection: it is very strong in the case of DPO, while it is reduced for the GPI and tends to disappear in the last case (GTS).

At present there are only two beef products in Italy that can proudly refer to EU recognition:

- The «Bresaola» of the Valtellina region, to which the GPI was attributed with the Reg. 1263/96 of July 1st 1996, published in the GUCE n. L 163 of July 2nd 1999;
- The «Vitellone Bianco» (White Breeds' Young Slaughter Bulls) of the Central Apennine region, to which the GPI was attributed with the Reg. 134/98 of January 20th 1998, published in the GUCE n. L 15 of January 21st 1998.

2. Labelling

Consumer information is one of the specific objectives of food legislation, even more so as leading or final objective of many regulations, *i.e.* those relevant to food products labelling, presentation and promotion.

Regarding beef, the current normative is indicated in Reg. 1760/00 of July 17th 2000 - abrogating Reg. 820/97 – that concerns the labelling of beef and beef products and creates a cattle identification and registration system. Such regulations arise from the market problems due to the first BSE crisis.

To identify and register cattle, Reg. 1760/00 foresees that every Member State develops its own system articulated as follows:

- Ear tag on each ear to identify each single animal, to be applied within 20 days from the birth of the animal and anyhow before the animal leaves the farm of birth;
- Computerized databases;
- Animal passports;
- Individual registers for each farm.

Every animal imported from a third country is identified in the farm of destination by means of an ear tag meeting the regulation, within 20 days of its arrival and anyhow before it leaves the farm. For each animal that receives an ear tag, the competent authority releases a passport that accompanies the animal's travels. In a similar way, the breeder must update the passports of the cattle present on his farm and keep an up-to-date register in which he notes all animal movements, births and deaths on the farm.

The labelling of beef and beef products has to involve the affixing of a label on each piece or pieces of meat or on the relevant packaging material, or for pre-confectioned products the appropriate written information must be visible to the consumer at selling.

The compulsory labelling system must permit to emphasize the link between, on one side, carcass, quarter or single cuts of meat identification and, on the other side, the single animal, or group of animals. This must be sufficient to permit verification of the information that appears on the label. The label should show the following indications:

a.) A reference number or code that shows the link between the meat and the animal or animals;

b.) The approval number of the slaughterhouse where the animal(s) were slaughtered and the reference to the Member State or third country where the slaughterhouse is situated. The indication must bear the words «*Slaughtered in [name of the Member State or of the third country] [approval number]* «;

c.) The approval number of the industrial unit where the carcass or group of carcasses was dissected and the Member State or third country in which the unit is situated. The indication must bear the words «*Dissected in [name of the Member State or of the third country] [number of approval]* «;

From January 1st 2002, the operators involved and the relevant organizations must indicate as well on the labels:

- The Member State or the third country of birth;
- The Member State or third country where the fattening took place;
- The Member State or third country where the slaughtering took place.

Nevertheless, if the beef comes from animals born, kept and slaughtered:

1) In the same Member State, can be indicated «*Origin: (name of the Member State)*» or;

2) in a same third country, can be indicated «*Origin (name of the third country)* «.

The operators and organizations that prepare minced beef must indicate on the label «*Prepared in [name of the Member State or of the third country]*» according to the place where the mincemeat was prepared, or «*Origin*» if the interested state(s) is not where the preparation took place. These operators or organizations can add to the minced beef label the preparation date of the mincemeat.

For labels showing indications different from those above mentioned, each operator or organization must submit for approval a disciplinary regulation note (regulation reference) to the competent authority of the Member State in which the beef production or commercialisation takes place. Besides, the competent authority can specify the disciplinary regulation (regulation reference) to be used by the relevant Member State, as long as this is not compulsory.

The disciplinary regulation note of the optional label must show:

- The information to be indicated on the label;
- The measures to adopt to guarantee the truthfulness of the information;

- The control system that will be applied in all the production and sales' phases, included the controls carried out by an independent organism recognized by the competent authority and decided upon by the operator or the organisation: such organisms should correspond to criteria indicated by the European regulation EN/45011;
- In case of an organization, the measures to adopt towards the members that violate the regulation.

The Member States have the ability to decide that the controls of the «independent organism» can be replaced by controls carried out by the «competent authority»; however the latter should have the qualified personnel and adequate resources suitable to carry out the necessary controls. The operator or organisation that apply the labelling system must sustain the control costs.

The disciplinary regulation note approval assumes that the competent authority confirms the correct and reliable operation of the labelling system, and particularly of the control system. The competent authority must refuse any note that does not guarantee the link between, on one side, the identification of the carcass, quarter or meat cuts and, on the other side, the single animal or animals, where it is sufficient to verify the information appearing on the label. Furthermore, any disciplinary regulation note that considers labels containing deceptive or unclear information is rejected.

If the beef production and/or sales is carried out in two or more Member States, the competent authority of these Member States examine and/or approve the presented note, always if the contained elements concern operations that take place in their respective territory. In this case, each involved Member State recognizes the approvals granted by the Member States in question.

3. Traceability

Traceability is an innovation of technical-organizational nature, a data collection and management technology to give information. ISO 8402 defines it as «*the capacity to find the history, the use or the location of an entity by means of recorded identification*». Regulation 178 of January 2002 of the European Parliament and of the Commission[2], relevant to the principles and general requirements of food legislation, establishes the European Authority for Food Safety and fixes the field procedures for food safety, it offers as well a definition with specific reference to food production. According to art. 3, comma 15, of this regulation, traceability is identified by the «*possibility to rebuild and follow the course of*

---

[2]GUCE n L. 31 of February 1ˢᵗ 2002, p.1.

a food, a fodder or an animal destined for food production, or of a substance destined or appropriate to be part of a food or a fodder through all the production, transformation and distribution phases».

In other words, we can assert that in the specific case of food products, traceability has the task of circulating information from each stage of the chain, from where they are produced and known (*i.e.,* agriculture, slaughterhouses, meat industry units), to the stages where they can be used (*i.e.,* distribution, consumers), and to have as well the information taking the opposite direction.

The traceability technology is therefore based on the capacity to manage harmoniously three specific functions of the information process:

1) The collection function - through appropriate recording procedures of the product's life - of the information that is requested from every enterprise that participates to the traceability program. This information allows to describe and know for every individual lot from the agricultural product: the parameters that influence the characteristics of food product specificity, the control procedures, the verifications and relevant results;

2) The transmission function to the other enterprises, interested in the traceability program of the necessary information, or of the information of a production disciplinary regulation note decided by all parts concerned;

3) The data management function: to consent that individual enterprises answer every request coming from customers (suppliers, enterprises buyers, final consumers) pertaining to information of the disciplinary. The traceability technology should allow a rapid and easy consultation of the gathered information through the right tools of choice and selection. This function must thus ensure the preservation and documentation of this information for all of the time required, depending on the nature of the products and for eventual legal obligations.

Obviously, these three functions can concretely be carried out only thanks to modern information technology. Because of this dependence of the effectiveness of its functions on information technologies, traceability requests that the food chain enterprises associate with technological partners specialized in information technologies that have the task of operating as an interface between the large computer and food chain offer enterprises. The specific activity of these enterprises is to operate as integrators-coordinators of the different processes that characterize the collection, transmission, storage and management of traceability through a global computer connection.

Besides, these technological advances have another task, which is not of technical nature, but nevertheless is very important for the success of the traceability process, since it satisfies two special requirements particularly necessary to the enterprises; to be carried out in an objective and reliable way and assure that their privacy be protected. They operate as mediators in the exchange of information between enterprises at the different stages, thus act as security agents («tiers de confiance»), since they are independent and guarantee the privacy of the exchanged information.

In last analysis, traceability in the field of food is today a particularly complex technology, because it results from the meeting of two important knowledgeable categories. The first is represented by the knowledge of the technical, economic and organizational itineraries of the production system and of the commercialisation of agricultural and food products. The second concerns the knowledge pertaining to the developments of computer technology and the management of information flow between enterprises located all along the chain.

There is a growing and serious interest in traceability technology by the Italian food production. The different points along the food chain show that traceability has gone beyond the stage of a fashion, being only the problem of few, or a simple bureaucratic link; it has acquired the full knowledge of being a necessity. Given the novelty of this technology, the approach followed in its adoption is in general still incomplete, imprecise, sometimes debatable, but in all cases constitutes an important segment of how deeply rooted is the sensibility to food safety problems in the consumers' thinking, and therefore of a more wholesome idea of quality.

It is still true though that the perception of the world of the real importance of traceability is still insufficient. There certainly exist important exceptions; but in general this technology suffers of a reductive interpretation leading to the exclusion of certain value elements that are the most important strategically and represent true results. This could lead to committing the mistake of overestimating its costs and underestimating its benefits.

In fact, traceability is not only a simple, though fundamental, instrument of food safety. It is not even a technology that is necessary to be adopted immediately under the pressure of worried consumers. Traceability is much more than this. With this new instrument should be pursued at least three different objectives:

1) To give greater transparency to the relation between production systems and consumers. The traceability thread represents the most important tool to invert the separating tendency between producers and consumers, that market globalisation always renders more obvious. Nutrition sociologists sustain that the main cause of the consumers' distrust and doubt is the actual increasing physical and psychological distance between the production system and the consumers. Therefore the traceability thread can be, before even a technical instrument of control, an instrument of reassurance and trust. This implicates that traceability must be the object of communication to the consumer, and therefore should be indicated on the label with a message or with an obvious mark which explains its significance and value;

2) Safety guarantee;

3) Base for whatever the control system might be; in fact no check system is really effective if at its base there isn't a complete and precise control of the materials. Obviously, to the traceability diagram should be adapted the management and certification systems of the ISO quality rules, the production disciplinaries, notes, HACCP, etc.

Traceability on its own is not a guarantee of safety, but is a tool that permits in the case of necessity to be able to intervene immediately and effectively.

Regulation 178/02, besides stating what is intended by «*risk*», «*risk analysis*», «*risk evaluation*» and «*risk management*» introduces the «*safety measure principle*»: «*If in specific circumstances, following the evaluation of available information, is identified the possibility of harmful effects to health, but there persists scientifically a situation of uncertainty, temporary risk management measures can be adopted to guarantee the high*

Image of cattle sector and its products

level of health protection that the EC pursues, while awaiting further scientific information for a more exhaustive risk evaluation. The adopted measures are proportional, and only take into consideration the commercial restrictions necessary to reach the high level of health protection requested by the Community, keeping into account the technical and economical accomplishment of other aspects, if pertinent. Such measures are re-examined within a reasonable period of time according to the nature of the identified life or health risk, and of the type of scientific information necessary to resolve the scientific situation of uncertainty and to realize a more exhaustive risk evaluation».

Consumers perception of cattle products: A statement from the Austrian point of view

J. A. Lederer

Department of Animal Production, Chamber of Agriculture,
Schwarzstrasse 19, A-5024 Salzburg

Summary

In Austria consumers expect, as consumers in all other European countries, a secure chain in all steps of production, processing and distribution and healthy products to low or at least to fair prices. But also they claim more and more a sustainable production system without negative impact on the environment. Therefore the first reaction on BSE-cases and the outbreak of FMD outside of GB was shock and uncertainty intensified by a broad public discussion in all media.

A dramatic decrease in demand for beef and further on a rapid decline in farm prices by 30% to 50% was the consequence, even there was no case of BSE or FMD in Austria.

To manage this crises existing strategies were improved. A central body of crises managers and decision makers, including representatives from the ministries of agriculture and health, veterinarian administration and the central cattle data base was established. State veterinarians in the field, employees of slaughter houses and advisors were trained for emergencies. This clear structure was extreme helpful to manage the false alarm in February 2001 but also in the first and only real case of BSE till now in December 2001.

The political impact of BSE and FMD and the public discussion caused by these critical problems in Austria will be:

- The financial support will be more and more dependent on farm size and production system (maintain smaller units, enlarge organic farming, etc.)
- For production clear and approved guidelines, controlled by independent authorities, will be necessary for defined products
- Strong regulations on animal welfare and animal health will be introduced

It is clear that this measures only can be realized in accordance with the EU-Commission but Austria still will work in this direction.

Image of cattle sector and its products

Riassunto

I consumatori austriaci, come tutti i consumatori della UE, si aspettano una catena di produzione , di trasformazione e distribuzione dei prodotti sicura e in grado di garantire prezzi più bassi o almeno equi. Richiedono, al contempo, un sistema di produzione sostenibile che non abbia impatti negartivi sull'ambiente. Tuttavia la prima reazione ai casi di Bse e di afta a di fuori del Regno Unito hanno avuto un effetto devastante sull'opinione pubblica.

Il repentino calo della domanda di carni bovine ha prodotto un riduzione dei prezzi alla fonte, stimabili fra il 30% e il 50%, anche se in Austria non si sono registrati casi di BSE o afta.

Per gestire la crisi, sono state rafforzate le misure vigenti. È stata istituita una unità di crisi composta da rappresentanti del Ministero della Agricoltura e della Sanità, enti veterinari ed è stato creato un banca dati centralizzata contenente i dati degli allevamenti bovini. Veterinari pubblici, organici dei mattatoi e supervisori sono stati preparati e formati per le emergenze. Questa struttura così snella ha permesso di affrontare con successo il falso allarme del Febbraio 2001 e l'unico caso reale di BSE documentato in Austria.

L'impatto politico della BSE e dell'afta e il dibattito pubblico sorto in seguito a questi rilevanti problemi hanno prodotto delle conseguenze che sono così sintetizzabili:

- In futuro, il supporto finanziario statale sarà sempre più in funzione della dimensione delle aziende e dei sistemi di produzione (mantenimento di aziende più piccole, sostegno all'agricoltura biologica).
- Sarà necessario definire delle linee guida (controllate da autorità indipendenti) applicate alla produzione zootecnica e e a quella di determinati prodotti.
- Saranno introdotte rigide regolamentazioni finalizzate al benessere e la salute degli animali.

Queste, ed ogni futura iniziativa, verranno ovviamente adottate in completo accordo con le direttive della UE.

1. Introduction

Consumers expect a secure chain in all steps of production, processing and distribution of food as well as healthy products to low or at least to fair prices. In addition they claim more and more a sustainable production systems without negative impact on the environment. Therefore the first reaction on BSE cases and the outbreak of FMD outside of UK was shock and uncertainty. The consequences were a dramatic decrease in demand for beef and further on a rapid decline of farm prices by 30% to 50% in most of the EU member countries. To manage this crises in Austria new strategies were developed and introduced.

2. Impact of BSE and FMD on the image of the cattle sector

The crises caused by BSE and FMD influenced the opinion of the consumers with regard to farm products in general significantly in a negative sense. At least in Austria a majority of the population to not longer believe production in big units, so called «industrial farming», can be handled by the farmers in a adequate and sure way. People are afraid heavy medical treatments of the animals cause residuals in the products and leads to growing resistances against antibiotics in human medicine.

The loss of confidence in cattle products, mainly in beef, led in a first reaction to a dramatic change in the human diets. Quite a big number of people cancelled completely beef and even other meat or at least reduced the consumption. Intensive information campaigns and advertising did not influence this behaviour very much. A slight recovery could be observed up to the end of the year 2001 but the consumption of beef per capita is still under the level of 2000.

3. Management of the crises

To manage this and further crises in food production caused by unexpected outbreaks of epidemics in a proper way existing strategies were improved. In Austria immediately after the first confirmed case of FMD on the continent a central body of so called crises managers was installed. This competent group of politicians and experts consists of representatives from the

- ministry of agriculture
- ministry of health and social affairs
- veterinarian administration
- central cattle data base

In regular and ad hoc meetings the actual situation in the country itself as well as abroad was judged and if necessary adequate measures are arranged.

A further responsible task of the group is information management and information policy. This centralized information system should avoid as far as possible false announcements and alarms and should also guarantee objective information for the society.

On the regional level responsible experts like

- state veterinarians in the districts and in the slaughter houses
- employees of the slaughter houses
- official advisors of the chamber of agriculture

were instructed and trained by the central body in all necessary specific measures in order to avoid a spreading of the epidemic.

In a checklist it is clear defined how it should proceed immediately after an epidemic outbreak. The main contents of such a checklist are:

- responsible persons
  - function
  - tasks
  - competences
  - address, telephone, fax, e-mail

Image of cattle sector and its products

- necessary information
  - source
  - farm data
    - location
    - type of farm
    - number and species of animals
    - neighbours
  - infected animal
    - ear tag number
    - date of birth
    - sex
    - breed
    - pedigree
    - origin
    - movements of the animal
  - feed stuff on the farm
    - type
    - producer
    - supplier

- verification of information

- information flow
  - to decision makers
  - from decision makers to
    - responsible persons in the field
    - the affected farmer
    - the media

An other important part of crises management is a clear understandable and comprehensive information of the farmers on the epidemic itself (first indications, typical symptoms, etc.) and how to react in case of an eventual outbreak in there herds in a proper and efficient way. At least a support program for farmers direct affected by the epidemic has to be established including not only financial but also psychological support.

4. Assessment of the political impact

In Austria there is a growing critic not on the European agricultural policy in general but on specific measures. It is claimed more and more that direct payments and premiums shout depend strictly on farm size and production systems favouring small units and organic farming.

In order to improve the confidence in cattle products approved guidelines for all steps in the production chain, with a clear documentation and controlled by independent authorities, are necessary. Therefore an agency for food safety is established by the ministries of agriculture and health affairs were all competences are concentrated.

How confidence in cattle products can be improved is demonstrated on the following guidelines of an Austrian beef product offered under the trademark «Salzburger Naturbeef» on the market:

- Type of cattle
  - beef or dual purpose breeds
  - young castrated males and females
  - castration at an age between 2 and 3 month
  - age at slaughter 7 to 10 month
- Feeding
  - suckling during the whole lactation period after birth
  - pasture during summer feeding
  - cereals as supplement during winter feeding
- Farming
  - consideration of the EU-guidelines for organic farming
  - high standards for animal welfare
  - verification by an official registered organisation
- Veterinarian control
  - obligate routine tests for specific epidemics
  - depending on the farm size 2 to 3 documented checks per year of the whole herd
- Quality standards of the product
  - high quality of the carcass in general
  - classification in E, U or R
  - fat class II or III

In the context with consumers perception animal welfare and animal health of farm animals can no longer be neglected because consumers are reacting more and more sensitive on problems in this field. Housing systems and especially transportation will therefore be regulated in future very strictly by the European Commission and by the national governments. In general this will be accepted by the farmers but it is important to have unique regulations in all EU member countries in order to have fair and equal conditions for all farmers of the common market.

Production and consumption in CEE countries in the light of EU integration: expectations and prospects

M. Zjalic[1], F. Habe[2] and S. Pistoni[1]

[1]European Association for Animal Production (EAAP), Via Nomentana 134,
00162 Rome, Italy
[2]Zootechnical Department, Biotechnical Faculty, Ljubljana, Slovenia

Summary

The paper deals with the production and consumption of cattle products in ten EU candidate countries from the Central and Eastern Europe. It also briefly reviews developments in the period 1993-99. The present situation is compared with the expected developments and in the light of the process of integration with the EU. In the past, cattle production and cattle products have always enjoyed a positive image. The cattle breeding was considered as the most natural transformation of plants that can not be consumed directly by humans in healthy and nutritious products. Production and consumption of cattle products declined sharply in the period of transition. The traditionally positive image of the sector has been marred by BSE crisis. Urbanisation, equal employment opportunities and declining share of food in the total family expenditure lead to an increase in consumption of convenience and cheaper animal products. The paper refers to a preliminary position of the European Commission regarding the implementation of some elements the Common Agricultural Policy in new Member States after the accession. Perspective of the sector after the accession to the European Union is an increase in demand, which will be met mainly by local production but an increase in net imports of milk and products and beef is expected in almost all EU candidate countries.

Key words: Central-Eastern Europe, EU enlargement, consumption and production, cattle, milk.

Riassunto

Il documento analizza le produzione e il consumo dei prodotti zootecnici nei dieci Paesi del dell'Europa centro orientale candidati all'ingresso nella UE. L'articolo propone una breve panoramica sugli sviluppi ottenuti nel periodo 1993-99. La situazione attuale è confrontata con le aspettative di sviluppo e nell'ottica di integrazione all'interno della UE. Nel passato, la produzione ed i prodotti bovini hanno sempre fornito una immagine positiva. L'allevamento bovino è stato considerato come il più naturale sistema per consumare vegetali e nutrienti altrimenti non commestibili. La produzione ed il consumo dei prodotti bovini è drasticamente diminuito nel periodo di transizione. La tradizionale immagine positiva del settore è stata affossata dalla crisi del BSE. La globalizzazione, l'applicazione delle pari opportunità e la diminuzione del consumo pro capite di carne all'interno delle famiglie hanno portato all'aumento della ricerca della convenienza e, quindi, di prodotti animali più economici. La relazione fa riferimento alle posizioni iniziale della Commissione Europea in merito all'implementazione di alcuni requisiti dettati dalla Politica Agricola Comunitaria per i paesi entranti. La prospettiva del settore dopo l'ingresso nella UE dei paesi dell'Europa centro-orientale prevede una crescita della domanda, che verrà soddisfatta principalmente dalla produzione locale, ma anche in una crescita della rete di importazione di latte, derivati e carni bovine dai Paesi della Comunità.

Parole chiave: Europa Centro-Orientale, allargamento della Comunità Europea, consumo e produzione, allevamenti bovini, latte.

1. Cattle inventory

The cattle inventories declined both in ten candidate countries and in the EU. In the period 1993-2001 (Table 1) the decline in the EU was much slower: from 84.9 to 82.3 millions or 4.1 percent compared with the decline from 21.1 to 14.2 millions or 32.6 percent in candidate countries. It should be noted that the decline varied among countries, with signals of stabilisation and even upturns (Slovenia) in the last two years. Inventories in the EU and CEECs cannot be compared. The milk and beef production in CEECs depends primarily on dual-purpose cattle breeds. Statistical data includes dairy cows and other animals with very low milk production. (Erjavec, 2000).

Table 1. Cattle inventories (in 1 000 heads).

	1993	2001
Bulgaria	974	640
Czech Republic	2 512	1 582
Estonia	615	253
Hungary	1 159	805
Latvia	1 144	367
Lithuania	1 701	748
Poland	7 643	5 734
Romania	3 683	2 965
Slovakia	1 203	646
Slovenia	504	494
CEEC	*21 138*	*14 234*
EU (15)	*84 905*	*82 319*

Source: FAOSTAST, 2002.

2. Milk

2.1. Milk production

In the period of social changes the milk production as well as all other branches of economy encountered structural, ownership and market changes. In the period 1993-2001, the milk production in EU was stabilised at the level of some 120 million tons. In Central and Eastern European countries, the initial sharp decline in milk production in the first years of transition has slowed down with an upturn trend in Romania, Hungary and Slovenia. The total milk production in ten candidate countries was around 28 million tons (Table 2).

Milk production in CEEC is characterised by low milk yield, which is, except for the Czech Republic and Hungary, at the levels reached in EU countries some 20 to 30 years ago. This is mainly due to the low genetic potential of dairy herds, inadequate nutrition and shortage of feed. In addition, the sector is affected by:
- inadequate milking technology and low quality of milk;
- shortage of capital for investment in technology improvements;
- insufficient managerial skills both in fields of technology and economy of production;

In countries with farm structures based on small units, it represents a basic element of the social safety net providing food and cash to poor farmers. (Habe *et al.*, 1998).

2.2. Milk consumption

In 1993, per capita milk consumption in CEEC varied between 48 percent (Bulgaria 157 kg) and 170 percent (Lithuania – 554 kg) of the consumption in EU (325 kg). Per capita consumption is obviously higher in countries with the longer tradition in relatively intensive

Table 2. Milk production (in 1 000 tons).

	1993	2001
Bulgaria	1 341	1 290
Czech Republic	3 454	2 708
Estonia	808	690
Hungary	2 080	2 143
Latvia	1 156	855
Lithuania	2 067	1 810
Poland	12 639	12 030
Romania	3 670	5 047
Slovakia	1 250	1 102
Slovenia	550	634
CEEC	*29 015*	*28 309*
EU (15)	*120 630*	*121 137*

Source: FAOSTAST, 2002.

milk production, such as Baltic countries and Poland, while it is much lower in Bulgaria, Romania and Hungary (Figure 1). However, it should be noted that in the period under the review, the milk consumption increased in Slovenia, Bulgaria and Romania.

In traditional rural societies, milk production used to have an ethic connotation: the first and basic food after the breast-feeding and an essential part of the diets of old and sick. For farmers, milk and milk products were the main sources of protein and energy in springs and early summers that, historically, were the critical periods of shortage of other foods. Fresh milk, home made yogurts, sour milk, cream, home made butter, cottage cheese, cheese in brine, hard cheese and even whey were a part of cuisine and diets all over the region. Each ethnical group has in its cultural heritage recipes for dishes containing milk and milk products. Sour cream (and, of course, paprika) represent a typical ingredient in many dishes of the famous Hungarian cuisine. More to the North and East - butter and cream are used in the preparation of meat, fish and vegetable dishes. Traditional cookies and pies cannot be imagined without milk, fresh or hard cheese and cream or butter. In recent decades, the growing popularity of the Mediterranean - Italian cuisine (pizzas and pastas, mainly) enlarged the forms of cheese consumption.

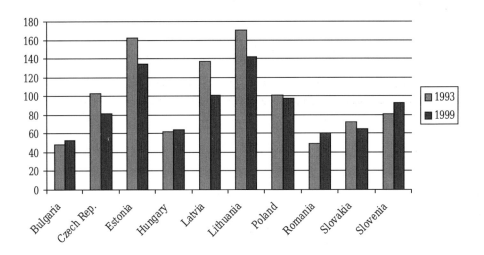

Figure 1. Index of per capita milk consumption (EU 15 = 100)
Source: FAOSTAT, 2002.

In the second half of the last century, urban population in the majority of CEEC had relatively high consumption of milk and milk products, mainly through various forms of catering (kindergardens, schools, and cantinas) and due to low, subsidised, prices. The total milk consumption sharply declined in the first years of transition, but in the period under the review, it is showing trends of stabilisation and, as shown above, a moderate growth in some countries. In countries where small family farms represent the basic structure, a part of the milk is used on farms for human consumption, for on farm processing, for sale at local markets and for feed.

Nutritional habits are in a process of continuous changes. In the first years of transition the introduction of imported diversified milk products such as milk drinks, processed soft cheese and creams, attracted good part of consumers. After the saturation of markets with imported exotic products and new products produced by local dairies (often owned by multinationals), a part of consumers is turning back to traditional local products, but now with much higher requirements for presentation, convenience, confection, composition (fat content). Major crises affecting the cattle sector in the late 90's did not have an impact on milk consumption in CEE countries.

2.3. EU Accession

In the current enlargement round, negotiations on chapter 7 (agriculture) have been opened with ten candidate countries. Assuming that ten new Member States could join the Union in 2004, the European Commission has elaborated scenarios and options regarding the application of the Common Agricultural Policy in new Member States. In general, it is expected that there will be no two-tier agricultural policy in the EU but one Common Agricultural Policy for all Member States. This does not exclude necessary transitional arrangements provided that they are in line with the relevant criteria of the application of the acquis as it stands at the moment of accession.

Despite efforts and – in most countries successful developments - restructuring of agriculture and food industries is still far from being complete, particularly in the livestock sector. The competitiveness of agriculture and the agro-food chain in the candidate countries is generally much lower than the EU average. The unfavourable farm structure in the candidate countries, i.e. in particular the large number of small farms and the existence of durable semi-subsistence farming combined with the presence of an emerging commercial farming sector pose a range of administrative and economic dilemmas for the Common Agricultural Policy. This dualism of structures is likely to exacerbate political tensions during the restructuring process, when not only farm structures but up and downstream infrastructure, services, and off-farm employment opportunities will require development.

Recent EU projections for the main commodities show that the candidate countries would be expected to somewhat increase their surplus production of cereals, oilseeds and pigmeat until 2006 (in a status quo scenario without accession). Milk and beef production would be expected to decline with many countries becoming net importers as consumer income and demand grows.

Image of cattle sector and its products

The effects of the application of EU price policy in the candidate countries will be to slightly positive on beef and dairy production are, but not enough to cause a significant increase compared to current production levels. The major impact of direct payments on production would be a faster development of specialised beef production, subject to the suckler cow premium ceilings.

As assessed by the Commission, a key risk during the early years after accession is that the restructuring process and Community instruments will be associated with growing rural unemployment and poverty without being able to tackle the root problem of alternative sources of income directly. In this respect, measures that undermine semi-subsistence farming and its welfare function could be counter-productive, particularly if no other safety net is available.

2.4. Direct payments

Direct payments are granted to farmers in EU-15 for a number of arable crops and cattle following the support price cuts of the 1992 and Agenda 2000 reform in these sectors. They will be extended to milk from 2005 onwards, in parallel to the support price cuts programmed for that sector.

In their negotiating positions on this issue, all candidate countries have requested that direct payments be granted to their farmers after accession to the same extent as farmers in the EU. In the negotiations the EU has not yet expressed a view on the issue, but stated that it will take a position at a later stage of the negotiations after a thorough examination of all the aspects related to the issue. For the time being, a draft position paper proposes that direct payments should be gradually introduced in the new Member States during a transition period. Such a phase is necessary to ensure the smooth integration of the candidate countries into the Common Agricultural Policy, while maximising the opportunity for the restructuring of their agricultural sector. The duration of that period should reflect the need to maintain sufficient incentives for restructuring: bringing semi-subsistence farms into the market, creating alternative jobs off-farm, and ensuring the competitiveness of the commercial sector. The positive effects of rural development, investment and structural funds programmes covering infrastructure, services and alternative rural employment require time. The effects of high direct payments would be immediate and negative. Ten years would appear necessary before the normal EU-level of direct payments should be reached. (European Commission, 2002)

It has been proposed that, in a first step, direct payments would be introduced in the new Member States equivalent to a level of 25% in 2004, 30% in 2005 and 35% in 2006 of the present system. In a second step after 2006, direct payments would be increased by percentage steps in such a way as to ensure that the new Member States reach in 2013 the support level then applicable.

2.5. Milk quotas

The milk quota regime is targeted at ensuring a balance between supply and demand on the dairy market. Through the regime dairy production is contained by restricting the production in each Member State to a national reference quantity that operates in combination with a dissuasive levy on milk produced in excess of quotas allocated to individual milk producers (additional levy). The national reference quantity is distributed between individual producers according to Community criteria and procedures.

As regards milk quotas and regional premium ceilings for beef the candidate countries have used rather heterogeneous justi-fi-cations for their quantitative negotiating requests, such as:

- remote reference periods in the past (pre-transition period);
- more recent periods with a margin for further development of production;
- unused production potentials or reasonable production levels.

On this issue it is the Commission's view that historical references far back in the past should not be accepted. This applies in particular to periods prior to the year 1990. Policies and general economic conditions in the second half of the 1980s were very different from those, which prevail today and will continue to prevail in the foreseeable future. Moreover, experience shows that the statistical data available from this period are often not complete and solid enough to be used for the sensitive purpose of quota fixing. In line with the approach to base quota fixing on recent reference production, it would be appropriate to use production figures on milk delivered and for direct sales for the years 1997-1999. The resulting average production data appear to reflect best the recent production situation in Candidate countries and would, in particular, even out fluctuations affecting particular countries at different times. (European Commission, 2002).

2.6. Dairy premia

From 2005, EU milk producers will receive *dairy premia*. The level of these premia is programmed to increase as market support is reduced. Although premia will be granted to producers on the basis of their individual reference quantities, the total sum of individual reference quantities eligible for premia cannot exceed the total national reference quantity for the quota year 1999/2000.

Introduction of dairy premia in new member nations would start at the same level as for all other types of direct payments in 2005, i.e. at 30% of the EU level in that year.

Entitlement to dairy premia from 2005 on should depend on implementation of the milk quota system, in particular on the allocation, by 31 March 2005, of milk quotas to individual producers.

2.7. Perspectives of milk production after accession

The introduction of milk quotas on the basis of the reference period 1997-99, for some of accession countries would mean reduction in the local production and increase in imports while the major part of countries will, at least in the first years after accession, increase the local milk production. The general trend after the introduction of milk quotas, also based on the developments experienced in the present EU Member countries (Kvapilik 1998) could be summarised as follows:
- the milk production will stagnate at the level of the reference period;
- number of dairy farms will decrease parallel with an increase in number of dairy cows per farm;
- milk quotas will stimulate intensification of production, changes in the breeding objectives and increase in milk yields;
- a number of dairy or dual purpose farms will have to be closed or converted to beef.

Future scenarios and developments in milk production systems will certainly include:
- improved genetic potential;
- redesigning production methods;
- improved milking technologies;
- improvements in farm management skills and practices. (Habe *et al.*, 1998)

Rural development policy, allocation of Community funds for the on and off farm job opportunities and conversion of small farms into viable production units would require:
- development of appropriate technologies and services (extension, A.I., input supply, marketing of products) for small commercial and subsistence dairy farmers;
- support to the development of small processing capacities for local products;
- provision of direct and indirect public support for attaining social and economic policy objectives in this field.

2.8. Perspectives of milk consumption after accession

Milk consumption will grow parallel with the «internationalisation» of nutritional habits and an enlarged presence of special products from the west European member states of the Union. The increase in the purchasing power of population – growth of per capita GDP – will have a marginal effect on the increase in milk consumption. However, differences between countries with regard to the per capita milk consumption will remain, at least to the extent they have remained among the present members of the EU.

Number of dairy plants will be sharply reduced. Some will have to be closed due to the low and non-economic capacity, others from technical reasons, mainly outdated technologies and high risks of contamination of products.

On the other hand, it could be expected that a part of consumers would turn back to traditional local products which would stimulate investments in small processing capacities at village or even farm levels.

Producers' associations will have to play an important role, particularly in the first phase of the EU membership, to ensure the maximal protection of interests of their members and to adjust both substance and methods of their activities in accordance with the new requirements.

3. Meat

3.1. Beef production

Before social changes, the beef production in CEEC was based exclusively on dual-purpose breeds. Culled cows and weaned calves are main sources of beef and veal. In addition, a part of production of young fattened cattle (10 to 12 months of age and 400 – 450 kg live weight) which were developed in the 60's and 70's in a part of Central Europe mainly for export, was sold to domestic markets.

The current situation in beef production candidate countries is characterised by:
- Continuous decline in the level of production;
- Inadequate nutrition, insufficient local production of feed and fodder crops;
- Temporary or chronic shortages of cereals and feed concentrates;
- Over-investment in housing facilities;
- Low profitability of operations;
- Low priority or disregard of etological and environmental aspects of operations.

3.2. Beef consumption

Before the social changes, the level of beef consumption in Hungary, Romania, Czechoslovakia, Poland, Bulgaria and Yugoslavia was 60 to 40 percent lower then in the European Union. The share of beef and veal in the total meat consumption varied between countries from around ten (Hungary) to twenty per cent (Romania, Czechoslovakia, Poland, Bulgaria, the former Yugoslavia). The traditional central and east European cuisine counts over 30 dishes based on beef and at least twice as much based on veal.

In the pre-transition period, the total beef consumption in then existing states (Poland, Hungary, Bulgaria and Romania) varied between 9 kg (Hungary) and 18 kg (Poland) representing 41 to 85 percent of per capita beef consumption in EU. In the period under the review, the total meat consumption increased in Estonia, Poland and Slovenia. Other countries (except Lithuania) had a decline from 10 to 15 percent. However, beef consumption declined both in countries with the growth in total meat consumption and in countries with decline in the total meat consumption. For example, in Estonia, it declined from 26.6 to 13.8 kg per capita or 50 per cent reducing the share of beef in the total meat consumption from 51 to 24 per cent. In Poland, beef consumption declined from 13.2 to 9 kg per capita, in Hungary from 10.2 to 6.2 kg, etc. (Table 3).

Table 3. Per capita meat consumption (kg/year) and percentage of beef in the total meat consumption.

	1993	2000			Beef (%)	
	Total	Beef	Total	Beef	1993	2000
Bulgaria	65.5	15.2	57.4	9.0	23	16
Czech Republic	94.5	20.7	73.5	11.6	22	16
Estonia	51.7	26.6	54.0	13.2	51	24
Hungary	93.2	10.2	92.2	6.2	11	7
Latvia	63.4	30.7	46.0	8.6[1]	48	19
Lithuania	63.9	35.3	49.9	17.5	55	35
Poland	73.6	13.2	70.7	9.0	18	13
Romania	90.2	11.0	48.7	8.8	18	18
Slovakia	77.2	17.3	57.4	9.2	22	16
Slovenia	86.9	26.6	90.0	23.0	31	26
EU 15	*86.2*	*21.4*	*88.9*	*20.3*	*25*	*23*

Source: FAOSTAT, 2002; Dr. Ulla Von Trietel, 2002
[1]Estimate by Zjalic, 2002.

Reasons for this decline are various:
- reduction in the average size of the family unit and leading to fewer traditional family meals;
- changing work patterns and full time employment among women with less time for meal preparation;
- nutritional and health considerations – leading in extreme cases to real obsession by cholesterofobia;
- lack of convenient products and poor marketing – beef is still considered as a raw material (Brini, 2001);
- high price in comparison with other meats, particularly poultry;
- BSE crisis.

3.3. EU accession

The beef sector will be exposed to major changes after the accession. The support measures will stimulate the specialised beef production with major impact on production systems, breeding policies and the organisation of the sector. The functional system of animal identification and registration is essential for the efficient implementation of the Common Agricultural Policy in this sector. (Scheiflinger, 2001).

3.4. Area payments

Beef sector (as well as other animal production sectors based on pastures) will be supported by the area payment for permanent pastures in the amount of Euro 350 per hectare for the 2005 and the subsequent calendar years. The Commission has proposed that for the new Member States, this payment be introduced gradually in the ten years period.

3.5. Headage

Following the Agenda 2000 reform, Member States may grant additional payments per head of male bovine animals (calves are excluded), suckler cows, dairy cows and heifers. For the current Member Sates, the global amounts have been established on the basis of the reference year 1995. The additional payments should be calculated on the basis of 65 Euros per tons of gross beef production (expressed as carcass weight), excluding calves and including the trade balance in live animals (exports less imports expressed as carcass weight). The Commission has proposed that the period 1998-2000 be used as the base for this payment in the new Member States, which will, in 2004, receive 25 percent of the amount approved for the existing Members.

3.6. Slaughter premium

Slaughter premiums have been applied since 1 January 2000 and are payable on bulls, steers, cows and heifers from the age of eight months and calves from one to seven months old and of a carcass weight of less than 160 kg. They are paid upon slaughtering or export to third countries. Ceilings have been established per Member State on the basis of slaughterings and exports registered in 1995. Where the national ceiling is exceeded, the premiums are reduced proportionately. The Commission has proposed that the period 1998-2000 be used as a reference period for new Members. Payments would be introduced gradually in the ten years period.

3.7. Special beef premium

Special premiums for male bovine animals are granted to maximum of 90 animals per holding annually. The premium is paid once in the life of each bull from the age of 9 months and twice in the life of each steer (at 9 and then 21 months). Where the number of bovine animals covered by premium applications exceeds the regional ceilings, the premium per producer is reduced proportionately.

The ceiling is calculated on the basis of the total number of bulls and steers over 9 months old. The premium was introduced in 1992 on the basis of historical data selected for each Member State. The period 1998-2000 has been proposed as the reference period for the new Members. As proposed by the Commission, payment to new Member states will reach the level of payments to the existing Members in ten years period.

3.8. Suckler cow premium

Animals eligible for the suckler-cow premiums are cows and heifers belonging to a meat breed or born of a cross with a meat breed, and belonging to a herd intended for rearing calves for meat production. From 1 January 2000 the number of premium rights of individual producers cannot exceed the number they held at 31 December 1999 and the sum of such rights must not exceed national ceilings.

When ceilings for suckler cow premia were first fixed in 1992, it was decided that each Member State could choose one from among the three most recent years for which data was available: 1990 – 1991 – 1992 (regulation 2066/92). During the last accession, the stated principle was to take the figures for suckler cows for 1993 and then to add on a margin to cover cows in herds with dairy quotas of less than 120 000 kg.

For the current candidate countries the Commission has proposed that the national ceilings should be calculated on the basis of the total number of cows and heifers in the 1998-2000 reference period which:
- belong to a meat breed or are born of a cross with a meat breed, and,
- belong to a herd intended for rearing calves for meat production.

The preliminary discussions on the application of the system to new Members focussed on the definition of beef cows, which in candidate countries differs from the one applied in the Union.

With regard to the number of cows to be covered by the suckler cow premia, the position of the Commission is that the number of suckler cow premia should be inversely proportional to the national milk quota. In other words, the ceiling for suckler cow premia should not be higher than the difference between the total number of cows and the total number of dairy cows (expressed as total milk quota divided by average yield cow).

3.9. Perspectives of beef production after accession

The beef production is expected to recover from the current low level. Cross-breeding with beef breeds which was a general practice in some countries, will continue. The expected reduction in number of dairy cows due to the increased per cow milk production and a consequent decline in availability of calves from dairy herds for beef production will lead to specialisation of producers and increased beef production from beef herds. This process started to develop in a number of CEE countries together with increased contribution of beef breeds and cow-calf operations to the total beef production.

The major factors that might influence the future developments in beef production in CEEC are the current beef consumption trends; consumers' perception regarding beef consumption and the production potential in these countries (breeds, feed resources). In addition, there are still uncertainties regarding the impact of the implementation of etological principles in beef production systems in CEE countries and regarding broader possibilities and constraints for calf-cow operation. For the group of CEE countries development of small scale beef farms could be of particular interest.

3.10. Beef processing

As only some ten percent of slaughter houses and processing plants meet the EU standards, the major part of them will have to be up-graded or closed. Their geographic distribution will be influenced both by technical and economic considerations and by the implementation of the EU norms regarding the transport of live animals.

It is expected that the standardisation of products (SEUROPE) and payments in accordance with the quality of products will have to be implemented in all countries. This will have a positive influence on the beef production (price - quality ratio, stimulation of quality products, better returns to producers) and consumption (improved image and the confidence in the product). (Treitel 2002).

3.11. Perspectives of beef consumption after accession

Beef consumption in the future EU members will, most likely, follow patterns of consumption in European Union of 15, with regional variations based on traditions and nutritional habits («pork eaters» versus «beef eaters»).

The growth of the per capita GNP (now varying from 30 per cent to 95 per cent of the EU-15 average) will have a positive influence on the total meat consumption. Beef sector will have to find its place in the new situation characterised by the higher purchasing power of consumers, but also with the richer offer of diversified meats and meat products.

In this respect, producers' associations will have to consider the introduction of new tasks and activities in providing services to their members. These may include:

- improving the public image of the sector through information campaigns, underlining health aspects and connection between the nature and the product;
- promotion of local traditional cuisine;
- technical improvements in beef processing and commercial presentation of beef and beef products (cuts, ready made and processed products, etc);
- introduction of meat labelling as guaranty of the health status of herds and individual animals;
- convenience products - development of new beef products for new types of consumption (catering, families, slow food, new fast food).

4. Concluding remarks

Authors of the paper wanted to draw attention to possible developments in the cattle sector after the accession and to indicate the main direction of activities to be carried out by producers' associations in new Members of the European Union. Each of our Project Partners as business representative organisations is a social partner in negotiations on terms of accession. After the accession, our Partners will develop new activities on the basis of local conditions and as the continuation of international co-operation among the present Partners. Such an approach will make their work more productive and beneficial to their members.

Recovery of consumption of cattle products, particularly of beef, is crucial for the economic position of producers. This can be achieved by joint efforts by both old and new Members of the Union, and both at national and at the EU levels. Working together in this field also represents an operational contribution to the smooth integration of the cattle sector of new Members in the EU, which is a basic objective of the BABROC Project.

5. Acknowledgements

The authors acknowledge the direct inputs and advice provided by Prof. J. Boyazoglu, Aristotle University, Tessaloniki, Greece, and Prof. E. Erjavec, University of Ljubljana, Slovenia.

References

Boyazoglu, J., 2001. EAAP at the crossroads. Guest Lecture; Hungarian Academy of Sciences (in press)

Brini F., 2001. Gli orientamenti del Marketing dei prodotti agroalimentari zootecnici nell'ambito dell'Unione Europea. Domzale, 19/03/2001.

Erjavec, E., 1997. The economic position of cattle, sheep and pigs in the farming systems of central and eastern European countries. Breeding strategies for cattle, sheep and pigs in eastern Europe, REU Technical Series 47, FAO, 1997. 21-34.

Erjavec, E.; 2001. The milk production in the central and eastern Europe and the enlargement of the European Union. Biotechnical Faculty, University of Ljubljana, Research Reports 31, 2001. 45-55.

FAO-REU Technical series 43. Task force on animal production in Central and East Europe. Evaluation report.

First Round Table on Livestock Production sector in Eastern Europe as affected by current changes. Budapest, 14-17 April 1991.

Fourth Round Table on Livestock Production sector in Eastern Europe as affected by current changes. Zagreb, 20-24 April 1994 (case study on Croatia).

Habe, F., Zjalic, M., Erjavec, E.; 1998. Restructuring of the livestock production in Central and eastern European countries and EAAP (49th EAAP Annual Meeting).

Second Round Table on Livestock Production sector in Eastern Europe as affected by current changes. Berlin, 19-22 January 1992 (case study on Eastern Germany).

Scheiflinger E., 2001. Bovine Database and Premium Payments. Domzale, 19/03/2001.

Third Round Table on Livestock Production sector in Eastern Europe as affected by current changes. Warsaw, 11-13 February 1993.

Treitel U. Von, 2002. Die Fleischwirtschaft in Mittel – und Osteuropa. Vortrag beim Workshop, «Zukünftiger Handel mit Vieh, Rindfleisch und Milch zwischen der Europäischen Union und Mittel- und Osteuropa» im Rahmen des Ost-West-Agrarforums,13/01/2002, Berlin.

Workshop on «Self-help Organizations in Livestock Production». Berlin, 16-20 January 1994.

Zjalic, M., Habe, F., Erjavec, E.; 2001. Situation and trends in milk and meat production in Central and Eastern Europe as a base for the assessment of protein feed requirements. Protein feed for animal production, EAAP Technical Series No. 1, 2001. 65-73.

Cattle sector and production image in the EU: The case of Italy

A. Nardone[1] and P.P. Fraddosio[2]

[1]Department of Animal Production, Tuscia University, Viterbo
[2]Italian Breeders' Association (AIA), Rome

Summary

The paper describes the Italian cattle farming, through its main demographic and genetic structural parameters; the breeding of livestock and the herd composition.

The relations among the production systems and the quality of the animal products were examined and different examples of traceability were taken in consideration to guarantee the authenticity of typical Italian products, both meat products and dairy products, in conformity with the EU and national normatives.

The actions taken by the Italian Breeders' Associations for the selection of cattle breeds, selection to genetically improve the quantity/quality production, were examined as well as the services that the Breeders Associations render within AIA, for the qualification and the valorisation of the products and also on behalf of third parties for the agro-industy component.

Furthermore the paper analyses the Italian editorial system relating to animal agriculture; both in the mass media and in the agricultural press. Particular attention was given to the communication media of AIA and those of the Breeders' Associations as well as the development of the Internet web.

Riassunto

Il presente lavoro descrive la bovinicoltura italiana attraverso i principali parametri strutturali, demografici e genetici delle popolazioni allevate e degli allevamenti.

Sono esaminate, inoltre, le relazioni tra sistema produttivo e qualità dei prodotti zootecnici e vengono presi in esame diversi esempi di tracciabilità per garantire l'autenticità dei prodotti tipici italiani sia di carni sia di prodotti lattiero caseari, in applicazione delle normative comunitarie e nazionali.

Sono presentate infine le azioni svolte dalla Associazioni degli Allevatori per la selezione delle razze bovine ai fini del miglioramento genetico per caratteri produttivi quanti-qualitativi e sono valutati i servizi che le Associazioni stesse svolgono in proprio con l'AIA per la qualificazione e la valorizzazione dei prodotti e in conto terzi per le strutture dell'agroindustria.

Image of cattle sector and its products

La relazione infine analizza il sistema editoriale italiano sia dei mass-media sia del settore agricolo. Attenzione particolare è rivolta ai mezzi di comunicazione dell'AIA e delle Associazioni degli Allevatori e allo sviluppo nell'impiego delle reti Internet.

1. Introduction

This paper discusses three fundamental aspects of cattle farming in Italy:
- Structure;
- The tools of products' qualification;
- Publication, information and promotion systems.

2. Structural aspects

2.1. Systems

In Italy are reared about 7,2 million cattle, mostly for dairy production (Figure 1).
Cattle breeding can be classified in six main production systems:
- Highly specialised milk production systems with primarily Holstein Friesian or Brown Alpine cattle with high production capacity;

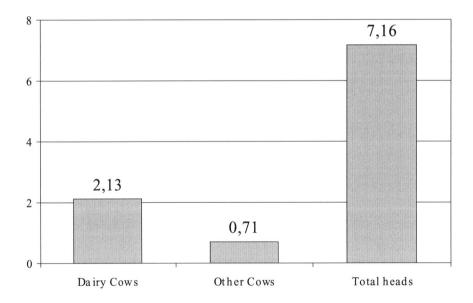

Figure 1. Cattle stock in Italy (million of heads).

- Systems specialised in dairy production that do not implement particularly advanced technical-management systems and use Holstein Friesian cattle of middle-high genetic value, or other dairy breeds with less production yield;
- «Local extension» dairy production systems that largely use native double purpose breeds (milk and meat) whose milk is mainly transformed into typical products;
- Systems specialised in meat production that according to the type of breed, age and slaughter weight produce:
  a) «Fattening white calves» of 220-250 kg live weight (mainly Holstein Friesian and Alpine Brown calves, coming from the national dairy herd and some imported calves that have already passed the colostrum period);
  b) Young beef breeds or crossbreed bulls (450-650 l.w.), mainly imported, and some of double purpose breeds.
- Semi-extensive (or semi-intensive) systems for meat production: mainly Italian breeds with a high production capacity (growth and yield) and excellent meat quality;
- Open-range systems for meat production with «local» breeds. This system exists only in certain areas and is rather limited.

The prevalence of milk production in Italian cattle breeding is evident when looking at the EU reality. In fact, in Italy there are 2.13 million dairy cows against 0.7 million for meat production. These numbers represent respectively 10% and 6% of the total respective populations in the European Union (Figure 2).

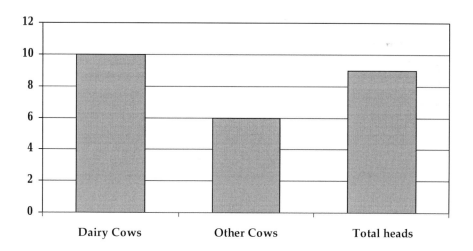

Figure. 2. Cattle stock (% Italy in Europe)

2.2. Farm sizes

Italian cattle breeding is characterised by the existence of many small farms: 48,3% of farms have less than 10 head (the corresponding average EU value is 22,5%), 37% have between 11 and 50 head (similar to the EU average, which is 36,8%) and only 14,6% have more than 50 heads (against 40,7% in the EU).
The animal distribution per farm-size category is as follows: 6,4% of all cattle is present in farms with less than 10 head (only 1,7% in the EU), 26,7% (against 15,6% in the EU) is present in farms with 11-50 head and 66,9% (similar to the average of 82,7% in the EU) of cattle are reared in stables with more than 50 head (Figure 3a and 3b)

2.3. Territorial distribution

Cattle breeding, especially dairy cattle, is mostly present in the north of the country. Cattle distribution on the national territory is related to the climatic and pedologic conditions.
   Dairy cows are in particular present in the Northwest and Northeast of the country; other types of cattle are more spread towards the South (Figure 4). Even beef cattle breeding is more present in the Northeast and Northwest of the country.

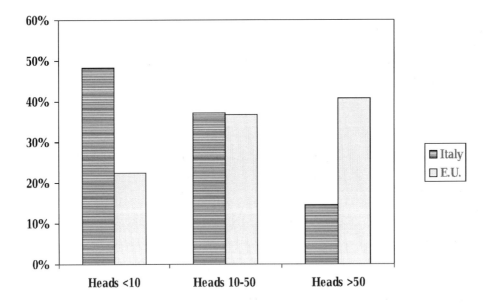

Figure 3a. Farm structure (% farm).

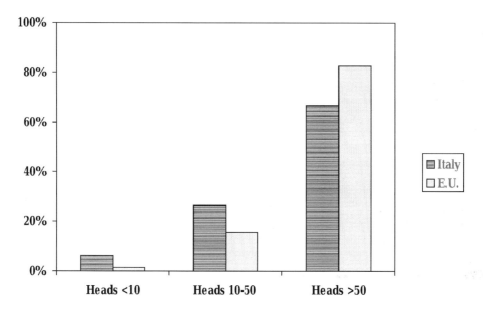

Figure 3b. Farm structure (% heads).

Fundamentally, milk cattle farm distribution is to be linked with the amount of water shortage for fodder growing. In fact, the less is the water deficit, the higher is the fodder production, and therefore the presence of dairy cattle; water deficit grows from North (218 mm H_2O) to South (700 mm H_2O) (Figure 5).

2.4. Ethnographic characteristics

The effect of the country's climatic and orographic conditions on the creation of the genetic types bred has determined, through time, a vast breed differentiation; in fact in the European context, Italy is one of the countries with the highest number of reared cattle breeds: 33 breeds, 14 of which are to be considered endangered. The greater incidence of the number of breeds in Italy is deducible from the ratio between number of breeds reared and number of animals. This ratio is equal to 4,6 and 3,6 breeds respectively in Italy and in the European Union per every million of animals reared (Figure 6).

The different genetic types with different production capacities facilitate the presence of cattle in the different environments that characterise the Italian territory. It is therefore necessary to preserve the different breeds, as to maintain a cattle-farming distribution capable of exploiting at its best natural resources, and to ensure human presence even in difficult environments.

49

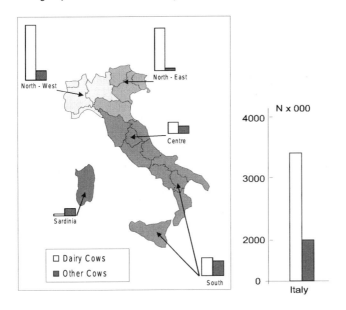

Figure 4. Number of dairy and other cows, in Italy.

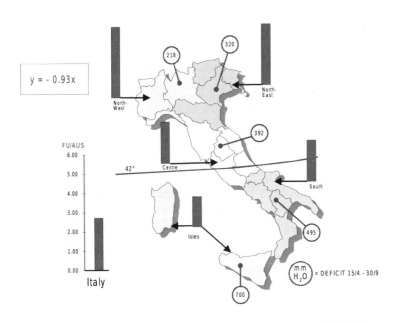

Figure 5. Forage production per ha (y) according to water deficit (x) per area.

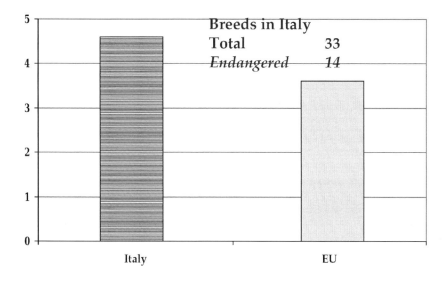

Figure 6. Structure of breeds; number of breeds/million of heads

During the second half of the **XX** century, at the beginning of the breeding systems' specialisation and intensification processes, Italian breeders took care of developing the selection of the most productive breeds, as well as maintained all the breeds that presented special attitudes for adaptation and/or production (Table 1). Today, this permits to obtain products of high value and standard, often linked to the breed and/or the territory, qualifying internationally the value of the Italian agro-industry.

The Gross Saleable Production (GSP) of beef for the year 2000 is equal to 3.406 MEURO, and that of cow's milk 3.793 MEURO. The sum represents 51% of the total Italian GSP of all animal products[1] (Figure 7a and 7b).

GPS (MEuro)	
BEEF	3.406
MILK	3.793
BEEF + MILK	7.199
TOTAL LIVESTOCK	13.917

Figure7a. Value of beef and milk on total livestock production value

---

[1]Beef GSP represents 24% and cow's milk 27%

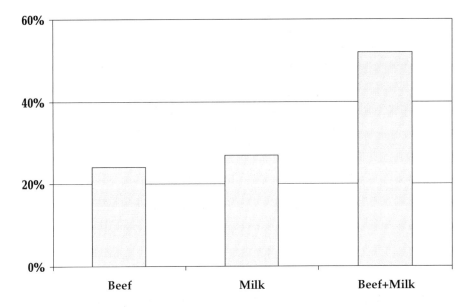

Figure 7b. Value of beef and milk on total livestock production value (% on total livestock gps)

3. Instruments for product qualification

The valorisation of products obtained from cattle farming should achieve different objectives:
- Consumer defence;
- Producer defence;
- Production system sustainability;
- Economic development;
- Biodiversity safeguard;
- Preservation of cultural traditions.

The products to sustain are:
- Food products: meat, milk and their derivates;
- Selected animals and their germplasm.

Table 1. Structure of the breeds

Frisona Italiana	2950000
Bruna Italiana	570000
Pezzata R. Italiana	300000
Piermontese	299000
Marchigiana	~55000
Chianina	~40000
Romagnola	14000
Rendena	Valdostane
Grigia Alpina	Pinzgauer
Maremmana	Modicana
Podolica	Sarda
Jersey and others	

3.1. Food products

The valorisation of food products is based on their qualitative characteristics; essentially, they are as follows (Nardone and Valfrè, 1999):
- Flavour;
- Authenticity;
- Safety;
- Salubrity;
- Technological quality.

Product *flavour* is always a crucial factor of choice for the consumer with a middle-high income.

Authenticity has an important value for the consumer because it brings to mind several positive images: to be natural, safe, typical and traditional.

Food *safety* is a pre-requisite (Codex Alimentarius in: http://www.codexalimentarius.net/; Aumaître, 1999). The consumer's attention towards this quality has increased in the last five years in relation to the onset of the well-known phenomena of BSE (Bovine Spongiform Encephalitis) or dioxin.

Only few consumers attribute value to *salubrity*. It is predictable that the increase in knowledge about the link between nutrition and health, particularly against cardio-vascular pathologies, allergies and immunity system defences, will determine an increasing interest in this qualitative character (Higgs, 2000; Kwak and Jukes, 2001; Nardone, 2002).

The *technological* features are aorticularly important for milk produced in Italy, as most of it is destined to the transformation industry.

Let's now examine certain valorisation aspects, specifically for milk and meat.

3.2. Meat

Regarding the *safety* of cattle products, Italy follows the EU regulations concerning animal health and food control. A demonstration of the good safety level of Italian cattle breeding systems is represented by the low incidence of BSE cases.

According to the OIE data (http://www.oie.int/eng/info/en_esbmonde.htm), in Italy the ratio (reported in 2001) between the number of positive BSE cases in cattle or carcasses of animals more than 24 months old, and the number of reared cattle, is equal to 14.1 cases per million head, against 189.6 in the UK, 128.5 in Portugal, 70.6 in Ireland, 24.8 in France and Spain and 19,0 in Germany. This is interesting as Italy imports large quantities of animal and cattle feed, and is therefore much more exposed to the possibility of contagion (Figure 8). Regarding the products' *authenticity, ad hoc* regulations establish specific rules:

- Two types of beef («Vitellone bianco dell'Apennino» - White young bull of the Apennines - and «Bresaola») have a «Protected Geographic Indication» (PGI) (in accordance with the EU Council Reg. N.2081/92) (Figure 9).
- Subsequent EU regulations have introduced precise rules for beef labelling to guarantee and protect the consumer (see Reg. of the European Parliament and Council n.1760/00 and the Commission Reg. n.1825/00).

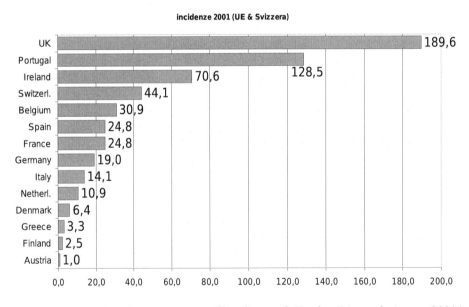

Figure 8. BSE risk evaluation. Cases /million livestock Heads > 24 months in year 2001 in UE and Switzerland (Source: Giuseppe Ru, DVM PhD Reference Centre for Animal Institute for Zooprophylaxis Turin, Italy).

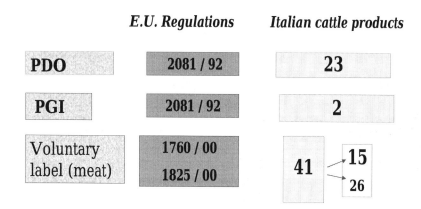

Figure 9. Elements to guarantee the authenticity.

Since the date of issue of the latter measures until today 34 voluntary labelling initiatives of beef and beef products have already been activated. Of these, 19 were activated in the slaughtering and distribution industry, and 15 were promoted by the agricultural world and the Breeders' Association systems.

Some of these are based on the valorisation of special valuable breeds, as in the case of the 5R (5R – «5 Razze» - means 5 breeds: Chianina, Marchigiana, Maremmana, Romagnola, Podolica). Others are based on specific animal nutrition and management «disciplinary regulations», followed during a specific breeding period, as in the case of the «Documented Meats», 'Zooquality» and «Conazo».

The labelling system promoted by AIA (Italian Breeders' Association) is interesting because it gives the possibility to the consumer to verify directly and immediately, at the moment of the purchase of the meat, the following items: the slaughtered animals' breed and category, and the farm and slaughterhouse of origin (Figures 10, 11, 12, 13 and 14). In synthesis, from the moment in which an animal is taken into a farm, the information of the subject (breed, date of birth, etc.) is transmitted to the Central Office. The latter, by means of a bar code on a smart card, sends to the farms labels that are applied on the registers as well as on the animal. These labels are retrieved at to the moment of the animal's slaughtering and affixed on each individual half carcass. When the half carcass is sectioned, exact copies of the label follow each individual cut. In this way the butcher, at the moment of the sale, can progressively account for the carcass weight. The weight of the carcass should be equal to the total quantity meat sold. The consumer can thus make the corresponding verifications with the data bank by means of computer systems, even connecting himself through a mobile phone.

Other examples of initiatives developed to increase the guarantee certification for the consumer are in experimentation:

Image of cattle sector and its products

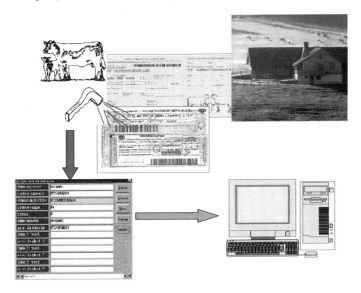

Figure 10. AIA's labelling system for the farm animal registration.

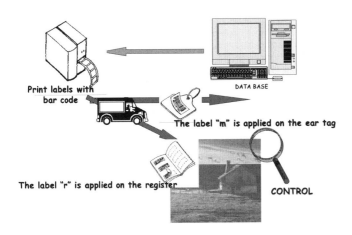

Figure. 11. AIA's labelling system in the farm label application.

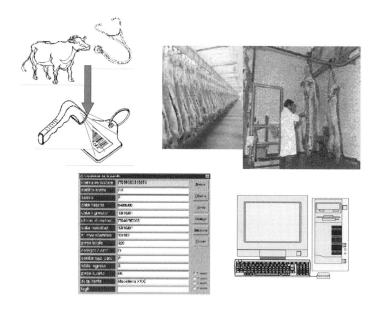

Figure 12. AIA's labelling system in the slaughterhouse.

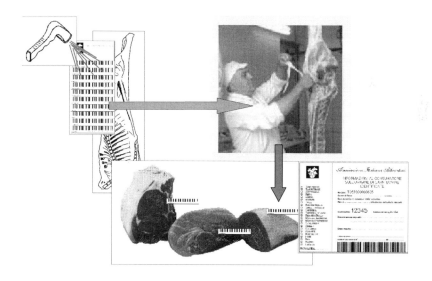

Figure 13. AIA's labelling system in the laboratory of dissection.

Image of cattle sector and its products

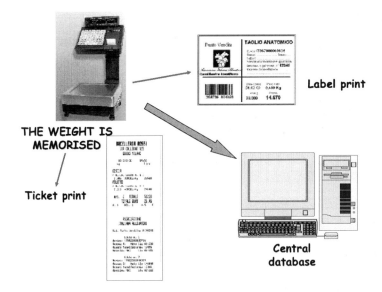

THE WEIGHT IS
MEMORISED

Label print

Ticket print

Central
database

Figure 14. AIA's labelling system in the laboratory of dissection.

- The Breeders' Association of Turin («Associazione Allevatori di Torino») promoted a plan of «genetic traceability» for the Piemontese breed; it should permit a DNA-test of authentication between DNA extracted from hair samples taken from the animals on the farm and the DNA extracted from the same animals' meat samples taken at selling;
- The Regional Breeders' Association of Veneto («Associazione Regionale Allevatori del Veneto»), through the work of its own analysis laboratory, promoted the implementation of an HACCP system (Hazard Analysis and Critical Control Points) aimed to ascertain the presence of meat or bone residues of animal origin in animal feed;
- Other examples are not reported for brevity.

3.3. Milk

A special interest is taken on by the activities carried out in Italy to guarantee cow's milk authenticity, quality, safety and technological features.

In Italy 23 cheeses have a «Denomination of Protected Origin» (DPO); there are 155 in all of the EU. About 11 million tons of milk produced annually are submitted to the control of public authorities (Local Health Companies and Zooprofilactic Institutes); these verify that the existing milk regulations are respected (EU Directive n.46/92 and DPR n 57/97). Beyond the control of the public authorities, there exist two other types of control:

- The first one is that of the milk's qualitative parameters to determine its commercial price. This type of control generally pertains to the protein and fat content, the somatic cells count, and the amount of bacteria and of inhibiting substances present. The control procedures and the involved laboratories are agreed upon between the *individual operator* interested in the dairy processing and the *producers*. The agreement determines the parameter limits to establish the final price of the milk. This system is spread across the whole territory. About 30% of these analyses are carried out in the laboratories of the Breeders' Associations – «Associazioni Allevatori».

- The second type of control is realised for the selection of milk breed sires. According to a national law, AIA is the authority responsible for the functional controls of milk production. AIA acts through the Provincial Breeders' Associations («Associazioni Provinciali Allevatori»), which employ official controllers for the field sampling. The data from the controls done by AIA are used for the progeny tests carried out by the National Associations, which always by law are responsible of sire selection. The data from the controls are also used for technical and administrative service assistance.

Every year, for these functional controls, about 11 million are carried out of tests to evaluate fat and protein content, and about 6 million of tests for somatic cell counts.

The Analysis System of the Breeders' Association disposes comprehensively of 26 regional or provincial laboratories and of a national «standard milk laboratory». The latter is officially recognised by the UNI EN CEI 17025 and the UNI EN ISO 9001: 2000.

The Laboratory standard provides to different functions: a) standardisation of 26 local laboratories, b) production of standard samples for instrumentation calibration, c) organisation of a «Proficiency test». Besides, it has contracts for the supply of various services for 78 dairy Industries and Co-.operatives, 26 Zooprofilactic Experimental Institutes, 13 Research Centres and 29 Private Laboratories.

The Breeders' Associations provide also assistance to Co-operatives that protect typical cheeses of special quality. For brevity let's only examine the case of the Parmigiano Reggiano. This cheese has a production area that comprises 5 provinces, in which comprehensively operate 563 dairies[2] with a production of more than 2.9 million of Parmigiano Reggiano pieces («wheels») obtained from 1.75 million of tons of milk, milked from 270 000 cows reared in more than 8 000 farms (Figure 15).

The help from the Breeders' Associations consists in technical support. The Parma Association, for example, actuates controls on qualitative and health parameters during production on the functionality of the milking machines, and on the correct management of the farms' technical regulations. The aforementioned control operations are carried out in respect to the production and guarantee protocol of Parmigiano Reggiano. The technical staff[3] realises every year 1950 livestock farm visits, 1 600 veterinary visits, 160 technological operations, and numerous verifications on the milking installations (Figure 16).

---

[2]The dairies are distributed as follows: Parma 215, Reggio Emilia 164, Modena 127, Bologna sn Reno 13, Mantova ds Po 44.
[3]Made up of 2 animal nutrition experts, 2 veterinarians, 1 dairy industry technician, 5 milking machines technical controllers, etc.

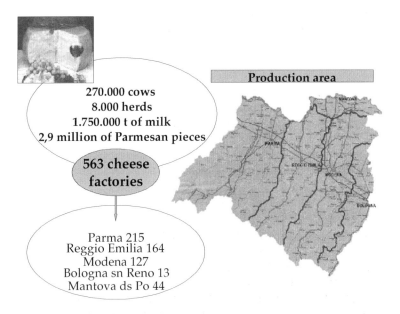

270.000 cows
8.000 herds
1.750.000 t of milk
2,9 million of Parmesan pieces

563 cheese factories

Parma 215
Reggio Emilia 164
Modena 127
Bologna sn Reno 13
Mantova ds Po 44

Production area

Figure 15. Parmigiano Reggiano

• 50 cheese factories associated for laboratory test
• 450 participating livestock farms
• 21 cheese factories with full assistance on the production chain
• 154 involved livestock farms

ACTIVITIES
• 1950 zootechnical visits
• 1600 veterinary visits
• 160 technological interventions
• 326 technical intervention relating to milking machine control

TECHNICIANS NUMBER

• 2 animal nutritionists
• 2 veterinaries
• 1 cheese factories technologist
• 5 technicians for milking machine control

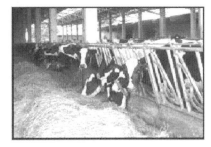

Figure 16. The example of Parma APA - Parmigiano Reggiano evaluation

The Breed Associations activate initiatives for cheese valorisation. For instance, the Alpine Brown cattle association has in course a project for milk standardisation in relation to its transformation.

4.3.1. Data-banks

The large amount of information available or accessible on farm level asks for a co-ordinated management of the data; for this objective AIA is building a computerised data-bank accessible by all those interested (Figure 17).

4.3.2. Genetic improvement

Amongst the basic actions for product qualification should also be included the services carried out by the genetic improvement system people for milk and beef cattle.

In Italy, are controlled about 1,2 million milk cows from different breeds for milk production (Table 2). The number of bulls annually submitted to progeny test are 564, of which about 62% belong to the Holstein Friesian breed. About 281 thousand beef cattle are registered in the Genealogical Books, belonging to the Piemontese, Chianina, Marchigiana, Romagnola, Charolais, Limousine, Maremmana and Podolica breeds.

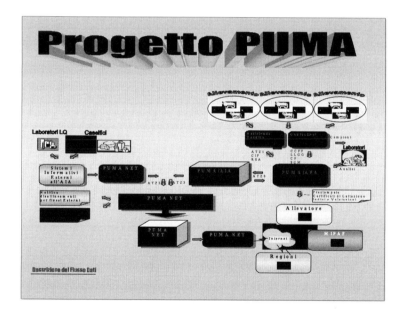

Figure 17. Computerised databank project of AIA.

Table 2. Milk recording, cows and herds, per breeds.

Breeds	Cows	Herds	Average lactation yield (kg)
Frisona I.	1 019 593	15 293	8 373
Bruna I.	135 682	10 550	6 010
Pezzata Rossa I.	45 157	4 178	5 734
Valdostana P.R.	13 369	1 153	3 404
Grigio Alpina	8 578	1 022	4 597
Castana	5 460	803	2 639
Jersey	4 601	460	5 165
Modicana	4 532	335	3 105
Rendena	3 876	214	4 505
Oropa P.R.	3 425	213	2 322
Cinisara	2 829	198	3 731
Valdostana P.N.	1 505	567	2 596
Pinzgau	1 050	107	5 590
Reggiana	840	120	5 353
Others			
Total	1 251 692	35 373	

The bulls submitted annually to performance tests are about 871. For some of the bulls are also carried out progeny tests.

The cattle fatherhood is ascertained by means of the «finger printing» technology, in a laboratory (LGS) managed directly by the Breeders' Association.

The genetic indexes formula varies from breed to breed (Figures 18, 19, 20 and 21) according to the production system, and in some cases also in relation to the environment and the breeding system (ANAFI, 2001; ANARB, 2001; ANABORAPI, 2001).

A consideration should be retained on the reason why in cattle a higher number of breeds is submitted to selection compared to other species. The greater dependence of cattle production systems on natural factors, and their stronger relationship with agronomic systems, requires cattle that are adapted to different environmental conditions and with different production capacities. Fundamentally, more populations are required, and each one must be selected for different objectives, to produce at its best in difficult breeding environment conditions. This choice is perfectly coherent with the biodiversity conservation and sustainability objectives. These objectives, although shared all over the world, are not always followed; cattle breeding has assiduously followed them in the last decades. As already indicated, animal genotype and production system diversity are important elements to obtain typical products and of special quality, giving an economical justification for breeding in areas that otherwise would be deprived of human presence, with the consequent problems of environmental degradation. A collaboration on these problematics between countries that participate to the BABROC project could be of great usefulness.

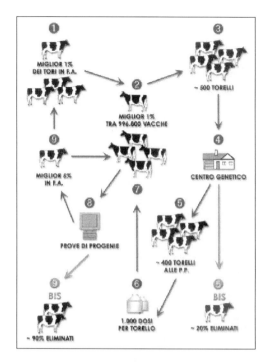

Figure 18. Selection schemes: milk production.

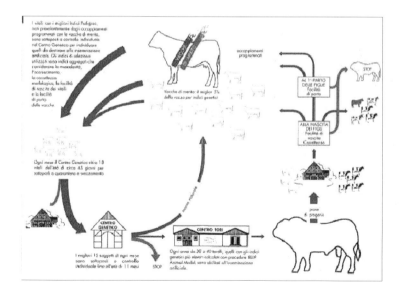

Figure 19. Selection schemes: beef production.

FRISONA	PFT
Kg grasso	0.47%
Kg proteine	1.99%
% grasso	10.82%
% proteine	37.58%
Tipo	5.69%
ICM	13.84%
IAP	9.11%
Longevità	9.11%
Cellule	11.39%

BRUNA	TEI (Total Economic Index)
kg grasso	1
kg proteine	3
% grasso	0,1
% proteine	0,4
Longevità	0,8
k-caseina: AA	0%; AB = 2,5%; BB = 5%

PIEMONTESE	Meat Index
Muscolosità	21%
Accrescimento	15%
Facilità nascita	43%
Facilità al parto	15%
Arti	6%
	Breeding Index
Facilità al parto	30%
Facilità nascita	20%
Muscolosità	25%
Accrescimento	18%
Arti	7%

Figure 20. Genetic index.

4. Publishing system and information

Product qualification or consumer defence policies can lack results if they are not supported by an adequate information system. To communicate in an efficient manner it is necessary to have professional preparation, valid documentation, timeliness of updating and intervention.

4.1. Who must be informed and of what

It is fundamental to establish exactly who must be informed, and what is the object of the information given. Producers, consumers and institutions are the three large categories to inform (Figure 22).

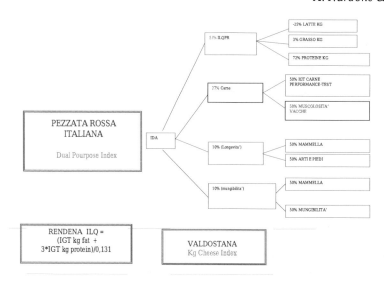

Figure 21. Genetic index.

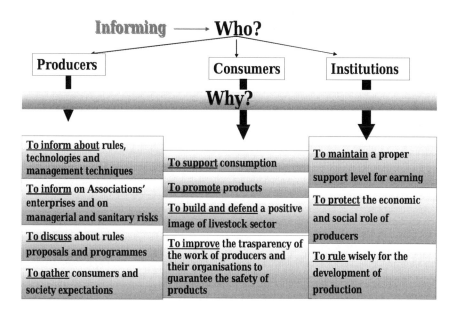

Figure 22. Who is to be informed and what about.

Image of cattle sector and its products

It is necessary to give to the producer clear and synthetic information on the technical and management innovations, on the health risks, on the quotations and market conditions. It is also necessary to involve him in the discussions and evaluations about proposals of new development programs of legislative measures. Correct information on the various features of the products must be given to the consumer, presenting them in a way that stimulates their consumption. The information reaching the consumer should give a positive image of animal production, improving the clarity between producer and consumer. The solicitations and elements reaching the institutions should permit to take measures that consent an orderly and sustainable development of animal production, protecting the breeders on economical and social level.

4.2. Information means

Useful cattle breeding information can be found at three levels: a) mass media, b) agriculture press, c) press specialised in cattle farming.
Mass media; in Italy there are (Figure 23 and 24) :
- different general agencies that present agriculture issues together with that of other areas;
- one radio and three television specialised programs;
- many daily papers that talk about national and local agricultural issues, with special communications that can be on a weekly basis.

Agriculture press; it can be classified as follows:
- About 50 national papers discuss cattle farming within the overall agriculture problematics (Figure 25).
- Eleven national press bureaus discuss agriculture issues; they are mainly present in the Ministries. There is also a printing agency (**AGRA PRESS**) specifically handling only for agriculture issues.
- Some papers/jurnals are specialised in animal production: a semi-monthly magazine («L'informatore zootecnico») and a series of bulletins discussing local animal production issues are managed by Regional and Provincial Associations. These present and discuss all animal production issues, and therefore also those of cattle farming and products.
- Cattle farming specialised press: it is almost always linked to the National Breeders' Associations that manage cattle genetic improvement. The purpose is always to inform the breeder about technical and economical matters and to maintain an open dialogue, to permit indications and requests to reach the field's administrative organisms (Figure 26 and 27).

In particular in the case of genetic improvement, there is an important information service for the breeder in choosing his breeding stock with specialised magazines such as «Cosa Valgono» – What are they worth - for the Holstein Friesian, «Indice Genetico Vacche» – Cow genetic index - and «Conoscere i Tori» – Know the bulls - for the Alpine Brown, «Büta Bin» for the Piemontese breed, etc. (Figure 28). These bulletins periodically indicate the sires' genetic values.

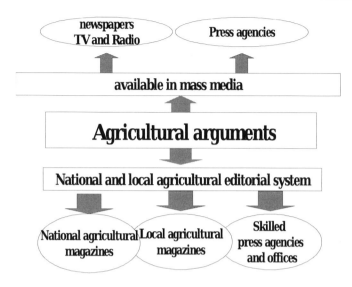

Figure 23. Information in the agricultural sector.

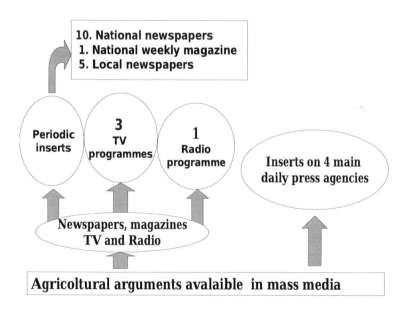

Figure 24. Agricoltural arguments avalaible in mass media.

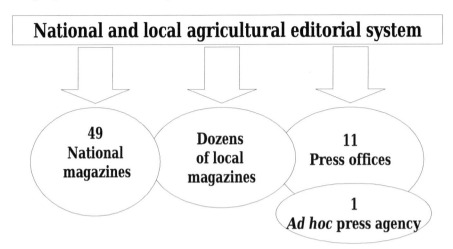

Figure 25. National and local agricultural editorial system.

Contents	Periodicity
Goals of the Association Technical and economical information Proposal and programmes Producers' helpline Information on expectation of consumers and society	Variable • 1 Fortnightly • 2 Monthly • 4 Bimonthly •1 Quarterly

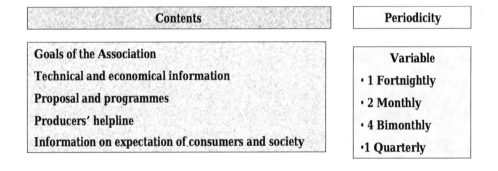

Figure 26. National magazines - Animal breeders associations (cattle).

Contents	Periodicity
•Goals of the Association •Technical and economical information •Producers' helpline •Proposal and programmes •Information on expectation of consumers and society	Generally monthly

Figure 27. Local magazines - Animal breeder associations.

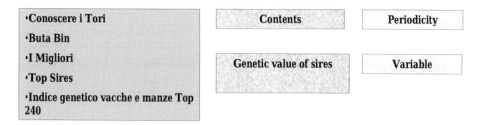

Figure 28. Technical references - Animal breeder associations (cattle).

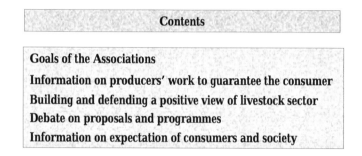

Figure 29. Press office of A.I.A.

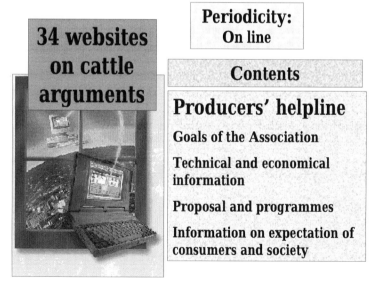

Figure 30. Internet websites - Animal breeder associations.

Image of cattle sector and its products

- Finally, AIA manages a newspaper called «*L'Allevatore*» – The Livestock Farmer - which carries out also the function of a press bureau. It is a kind of interface between the *mass media* and the *specialised press*, so that the animal production issues reach the consumers, government authority and political power (Figure 29).

4.3. Computerised systems

Another information task is carried out by the computer systems of the Breeders'Associations. The Breeders' Organisms are, since a few years, actively managing *web sites* specific for cattle farming, in which the breeders can find information relevant to the Association to which they belong, as well as the results from the genetic tests (Figure 30). This information tool is in rapid development for animal production.

5. Conclusion

Communication is essential in a world that tends always more towards market globalization, that speeds up exchanges and breaks down barriers, provided that it is correct and timely. This permits to reward the best, not to repeat fruitlessly experiences already done by others, and to transfer quickly all new information; in this way the technological, production systems and market evolution can evolve in an orderly manner and in line with the requirements or the preferences of the consumer and society's lifestyles, and in respect of the environment.

There is an increasing requirement for an horizontal collaboration between groups involved in the same issues (research, formation, production, services, market, information, etc.) and of a vertical collaboration between groups that take care of different aspects of the same problem (sustainability, traceability, quality, selection, etc.) or of the same product. This requirement is felt at country level and even more so on international level.

These are the reasons why it would be opportune to create for the BABROC project countries (Central Eastern Europe) an international network about the technical-organisational animal production issues, and about product qualification and its promotion; in this way the interaction between authorities, researchers, technicians and breeders would become an automatic action.

6. Acknowledgements

We thank the managers and the technicians of the National, Regional and Provincial Associations for the big amount of information supplied for this paper.

Reference list

ANABORAPI, 2001. Büta Bin.

ANAFI, 2001. Cosa valgono.

ANARB, 2001. Conoscere I Tori.

ANARB, 2001. Indice Genetico Vacche.

Aumaître A. 1999. Quality and safety of animal products. Livest. Prod. Sci. 59: 113-124.

Higgs J.D. 2000. The changing nature of red meat: 20 years of improving nutritional quality. Trends in Food Sci. & Technology 11: 85-95.

Kwak No-S. and Jukes D.J. 2001. Functional foods. Part 2: the impact on current regulatory terminology. Food Control 12: 109-117.

Nardone A. and Valfrè F., 1999. Effects of changing production methods on quality of meat, milk and eggs. Livest. Prod. Sci. 59: 165-182.

Nardone A. 2002. Evolution of livestock production and quality of animal products. Proceedings of 39th Annual Meeting of the Brazilian Society of Animal Science, Brazil, 29th July-2nd August

Conclusions by AIA's Vice-Chairman, Giuseppe Pantaleoni

Thank you and good afternoon; I would like to welcome you all on behalf of the Italian Breeders Association (AIA).

My task today consists in summarising the highly interesting papers presented during this morning's session, thus introducing the topics that will be dealt with in this afternoon's plenary session which will include, among others, the presentation of two interesting papers.

In this morning's session, three presentations were made, which I shall summarise in the order they were delivered.

The first presentation was made by Mr Claus, from Germany, who illustrated the situation of the cattle register systems adopted in the various EU Countries. The topic was therefore cattle and cattle breeding. From the above mentioned paper what emerged is that, if no register is in place, there is no room for policies, both as far as health aspects are concerned, and from the marketing standpoint, and as far as the funding provided by the EU to the beef cattle raising sector is concerned.

The history of the various cattle register systems that were adopted over time was illustrated, until the present day, focusing on the establishment of a single cattle register common to all European Union countries, making it possible to make a census of the overall European cattle population.

The second presentation was made by Professor Pieri, who started from the issues linked to the cattle register to illustrate all the activities that originate from it, from product traceability, to the definition of PGI (Protected Geographical Indication), PDO (Protected Denomination of Origin), i.e. to all those production rules allowing cattle breeding to achieve certified quality.

It is clear that traceability or traking alone cannot guarantee quality, but are simply, as stressed by Professor Pieri, a set of information for further use. Information must not overburden consumers, it must not come to be perceived as a saga written on a t-bone steak, as this would cause in consumers a harmful confusion. On the contrary, information must represent the basis from which to extract all the elements capable of reassuring consumers on the actual features of the product purchased.

In the Italian and European markets it is today virtually unthinkable to produce beef without availing oneself of a complete traceability project, guaranteeing the possibility to trace back all production phases.

The third presentation, held by Professor Lederer, from Austria, illustrated the image currently perceived of the sector, also as a consequence of the way in which the emergencies occurred in the past few years in the EU were handled (both health emergencies, and those linked to food safety). We can state that we must ensure we are capable of preventing these crises by foreseeing what could happen.

Image of cattle sector and its products

It is quite clear, underscored Professor Lederer, that the press and communication media have played an important role in the management of these crises: with special reference to consumer information, it should not be allowed to cause panic among the population by using communication in an incorrect manner. However, we must bear in mind that consumers have and want more information, want to be reassured with facts on what they eat. Information must not be a mere shield or weapon to counter the consequences produced by these crises, but must be something more complete, continuing, always and constantly there. At the end of these interesting presentations a debate was started.

We may say that all the three presentations highlighted the central role played by communication, in other words the importance of communicating in a better way compared to what we do today. A number of examples on the way these emergencies were managed in other countries were illustrated, such as in France, where authoritative bodies in charge of communication (also scientific) on beef have been established.

In this connection it was highlighted that two preconditions are required in order to provide real information: authoritativeness and truthfulness.

The role played in this connection by the press, both the specialised one and that meant for the greater public, must ensure correct and complete information, and may only be provided by means of a real inter-profession. The latter enhances the role of all sector's operators and not only that of the production world. Today debate is only open among producers, but we must consider what is upstream and downstream of this world, and act so as to establish a real inter-profession in the beef sector. This is the direction followed by Italian operators, who are trying to establish a real inter-professional structure which will no doubt make it possible to delve deeper into and solve problems common to the entire sector.

Crisis management» is another essential point in the debate. Special attention should be focused on prevention: epizootic diseases are there, always have been, and, unfortunately, we cannot be sure that they will not be there in the future. We must therefore plan the management of crises that may emerge in the future.

Many other aspects were made the object of debate: for instance the fact that for years our continent has been marked by changes in eating habits. We may for instance refer to the need for fast food services, to the fact that less people eat at home, that there is less time to cook, all elements that have played a part in partially changing eating habits. In percentage, today the consumption of white meat has increased compared to a few years ago, because in consumers' perception this type of meat is easier and faster to prepare, and costs less, an aspect that should not be downplayed.

All these changes have been noticed. However, these differences are far from identical in all European countries; not everybody has the same kind of approach, or the same problems: also applicant countries are marked by different situations in terms of these aspects. Therefore approaches, and the subsequent solutions, both as far as communication is concerned, and in terms of nutritional and food habits, and with reference to production systems, will necessarily have to be diversified depending on the various situations to be dealt with. Solutions must not and cannot be the same for one and all, nor can they be confined within the administrative boundaries of a State, as soil, climate, and mountain conditions may differ considerably within the same country.

In conclusion, we may summarise that we need mutual information, much greater than what is currently being proposed by the European Union to the applicant countries. Indeed, there is the need for a mutual exchange of information on conditions and initiatives implemented, with the aim of helping applicant countries to enter the EU in a coordinated manner, capable of answering current requirements. It is unrealistic to think that we may go on adopting individual actions, because the issues to be dealt with are so important, so full of meaning and topical, that debate on them cannot but be permanent.